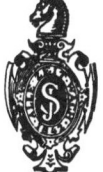

Recent Results in Cancer Research

Fortschritte der Krebsforschung

Progrès dans les recherches sur le cancer

32

Edited by

Springer-Verlag Berlin Heidelberg GmbH 1970

Robert S. Nelson

Endoscopy
in Gastric Cancer

With 66 Figures, 60 of these in Color

Springer-Verlag Berlin Heidelberg GmbH 1970

ROBERT S. NELSON, Professor of Medicine, Chief, Gastroenterology Service,
University of Texas, M.D. Anderson Hospital, Houston, TX/USA

Sponsored by the Swiss League against Cancer

ISBN 978-3-662-11671-5   ISBN 978-3-662-11669-2 (eBook)
DOI 10.1007/978-3-662-11669-2

Title No. 3647

To my Wife Mary

Foreword

Gastroscopy, the endoscopic examination of the interior of the stomach, has finally come of age. Although beset with multiple difficulties, and slow to develop, the method has achieved a sudden flowering in the past 10 years found in few other types of examination of the living human. The advances, the results of great interest and perseverance by many workers in all parts of the world, have been based on the happy combination of these efforts and the rapidly changing manufacture of various instruments to visualize, photograph, and biopsy all parts of the stomach at will. So rapid have been these advances that it has been difficult even for those intimately involved to keep abreast of the changes. The general physician public is in consequence still in considerable ignorance of what is now endoscopically available for the diagnosis of gastric disease.

Many interesting types of gastric pathology have been and are still being better defined by endoscopy, but its particular value lies in the diagnosis of malignant neoplasia of the stomach. Whereas in the immediate past it was necessary to restrict examination to roentgenograms, at best an indirect means, it is now possible to visualize lesions, photograph them in color, and biopsy all suspicious areas with great accuracy. A visual and histologic diagnosis of cancer of the stomach may be made in well-equipped institutions in an hour or less. Endoscopists are understandably eager to get on with the work, expand the employment of endoscopy, and diagnose gastric cancer in an early stage in ever-increasing numbers. These dreams lack realization because of numerous intangible factors, varying in different parts of the world, which still delay maximum use of the method.

The purpose of the present monograph is to briefly summarize the past work in endoscopy of gastric cancer, explain more fully the recent developments and their practical application, and to attempt to rationalize plans for the future. The author is not alone in this endeavor. Workers all over the world, many of them friends or former students, have helped to provide the information and crystallize the conclusions expressed. The American Society for Gastrointestinal Endoscopy, its counterparts in many countries, and international meetings such as the First Congress of the International Society of Endoscopy have aided immeasurably in disseminating information on endoscopy, particularly as it applies to stomach cancer. These exchanges of ideas and information, as much as the development of instruments and methods, are responsible for the recent realization of the dreams of all older endoscopists—the gross identification, visual representation, and histologic proof of gastric cancer. It is not difficult to see why those who have labored with this problem for 20 years or more are now so enthusiastic, and why we are anxious, if it is possible, to convince medicine in general of the advantages of early endoscopy.

But the practical aspects of any work, no matter how enthusiastically undertaken, cannot be denied. The literature is full of reminders that endoscopy needs a great deal of supporting evidence, as well as a lot of salesmanship, if it is to be efficiently employed. So, on to the facts which we hope will demonstrate clearly the true status of this method in the management of gastric cancer, and to the hope that they will be critically read and accepted.

The writing of any monograph is essentially a compendium of the help of many others, as well as individual effort. This work could not have been completed without the support of CLIFTON D. HOWE, M.D., who encouraged all its ramifications, FRANK L. LANZA, M.D. and BUNTWAL SOMAYAJI, M. D., my enthusiastic assistants in endoscopy, LOUISE KLARQUIST, who spent many hours preparing the manuscript, and the Olympus Corporation of America, who made possible the publication of the gastroscopic photographs, all taken with the gastrocamera.

Contents

Chapter 1

Endoscopy of the Stomach

History

A short consideration of the history of gastroscopy is useful to emphasize the difficulties encountered, the rather gradual development over a period of years, and the final somewhat explosive nature of the breakthroughs associated with this diagnostic method. No attempt will be made to give a detailed account of the evolution of the gastroscope. SCHINDLER (1950), who may be justly called the father of gastroscopy, has given an intimate and personal account well worth reading, as have others (WALK, 1966). Gastroscopic history may be logically divided into three periods: 1) early, during which various physicians made sporadic attempts to peer into the esophagus and stomach with poorly lighted tubes, with increasing success, 2) intermediate, beginning with the first partly flexible gastroscope, and 3) modern, marked by the development of all types of completely flexible fiberoptic endoscopes.

Early Period. The first determined trials to observe the interior of the stomach made a little over 100 years ago were with a straight, rigid, metal instrument lighted proximally by a lamp. A sword swallower was the subject, and the attempt unsuccessful due to poor illumination (KUSSMAUL, 1868). Another attempt was made, again unsuccessfully, but using electric lighting of a primitive type in 1879. In 1881 the first practical observations were made in the stomach through a rigid, curved, instrument, but again the method was discarded because of technical difficulties (MIKULICZ, 1881). Based on SCHINDLER's account, the period of 1881—1932 was active but discouraging, numerous types of instruments being tried, some rigid, some bent, some capable of being straightened after insertion, some open and some closed tubes with a separate optical system. SCHINDLER entered the field in 1920, and was greatly encouraged by what he could observe through a rigid gastroscope developed by ELSNER. His work with this instrument inspired him to construct one of his own, and in 1923 to publish numerous papers (SCHINDLER, 1923, 1924).

From 1923 until 1932, SCHINDLER, as well as others (HENNING, 1931, MOUTIER, 1932), accumulated gastroscopic observations with the rigid instrument. During this period, some excellent descriptions of gastric pathology were compiled, but once again the method began to fall into disrepute because of two factors: inability to adequately view the lower part of the stomach in many patients, and gastroscopic accidents, consisting of esophageal perforations for the most part. Although some endoscopists had very few of the latter, there were enough reported that workers advocated abandonment of the procedure. Regardless of danger, it was plain to most gastroscopists that the instruments then in use would have to be improved to allow better viewing and increased safety. This objective was finally achieved.

Intermediate Period. From 1928 to 1932 SCHINDLER worked with G. WOLF, an instrument maker, to produce a gastroscope with a closed system of glass lenses which would allow the lower end of the instrument to be bent to conform to the contours of the esophagus and stomach, at the same time giving good vision. These efforts were consummated in 1932 with the development of a straight instrument with a short metal portion connected to a flexible tube containing lenses for transmission of the image even when bent. This gastroscope proved extremely useful, allowing good observation of most of the stomach with a minimum of accidents, although these still occurred (SCHINDLER, 1933).

The improvement in the instrument was shortly followed by a much wider use of gastroscopy. SCHINDLER trained many men from all over the world, who in turn trained others. Other established gastroscopists obtained the new gastroscope and trained their share. Enthusiasm among endoscopists reached new heights, and knowledge of gross gastric findings increased. Good as the new instrument was, it became evident after a time that it, too, could be improved. Experienced endoscopists began to have doubts as to their ability to view the entire antrum, and realized fully that, because the instrument was so close to the posterior wall of the stomach, they could not often inspect this portion of the organ, or the area immediately around the cardio-esophageal junction. As might be expected, modifications of SCHINDLER's instrument were devised to correct these difficulties. An ingenious arrangement of one such modification was the addition of pull-wires to move the flexible portion of the gastroscope away from the posterior wall, (Eder-Palmer, Herman Taylor gastroscope) and addition of a chamber enclosing the objective lens, mirror and lamp to illuminate the mucosa close to the tip (Eder-Palmer gastroscope, Bernstein modification). These additions did help, but did not solve visualization of the antrum, even when the flexible portion was lengthened. A number of suction and forceps biopsy devices, attached to and incorporated within the gastroscope, were evaluated with little success (these will be discussed in more detail in Chapter 2). Several photographic modifications, with first tungsten and then flash lighting, utilizing reflex cameras attached to the eyepiece of the instrument, were developed (Chapter 2).

The net result of all this experimentation was considerable satisfaction with the ability to visualize the gastric interior, but nagging frustrations in observation continued to creep in, as well as the realization that the gross appearance of the interior of the stomach did not, in all cases, reflect exactly what was occurring under the mucosa. It became obvious that the new-found ability to photograph gastric pathology could be improved, that all areas of the stomach should be viewed, and the histologic documentation of pathology, especially in gastritis, ulcer, and cancer would be necessary to fulfill the potential of gastroscopy.

Modern Period. Beginning in 1958, gastroscopy was revolutionized by fiberoptics. How completely, and how rapidly this transformation came about can be realized only by the older, more experienced endoscopists who had been laboring in this field for the past 20 or so years. Suddenly, it was possible to view the antrum, pylorus, the posterior wall and cardio-esophageal junction, and occasionally part of the duodenum with great regularity. Not so suddenly, but just as reliably, biopsies were taken under direct vision of small lesions or areas, and beautiful, clear-cut photographs in color obtained of any area of the stomach. Although this took place within a relatively short span, a good deal of work and experiment went into the final production. The rapidity of the change confused even some experienced endoscopists, and a more detailed account of this era is probably in order.

Two instruments, both largely developed within the past 12 years, have been mainly responsible for the present impact of endoscopy on the diagnosis and treatment of gastric cancer. These are the gastrocamera and the fiberscope. The former allowed the average endoscopist to present his findings for review as final proof of what can be seen at endoscopy, and, in some cases, to make a diagnosis without prior endoscopy. The latter has made possible the routine examination of the entire stomach surface, and, with the modification for directed biopsy, histologic proof of the gross diagnosis.

It is interesting that the formal introduction of both these instruments occurred at the same time, at the World Congress of Gastroenterology in 1958. Both had been developed prior to that date, but large-scale clinical use was yet to come. At that meeting, TASAKA and ASHIZAWA (1958) presented some excellent photographs taken with the gastrocamera, and HIRSCHOWITZ et al. (1958) demonstrated the fiberscope. The acceptance and clinical trial of both instruments with expansion to all areas of the world has been remarkably rapid, but the full impact of these diagnostic aids has yet to be felt.

The idea of an intragastric camera and a workable instrument were first described by LANGE and MELTZING (1898), and, although technical problems eventually led to the abandonment of the project, some recognizable black and white photographs were obtained. A later intragastric camera, the gastrophotor (HEILPERN and PORGES, 1930), was developed which took fair black and white photographs, employing for the first time a flash bulb. This instrument never achieved widespread use. Eventually, Japanese workers (UJI, 1952) built a gastrocamera which, although beset with considerable technical difficulties, was eventually improved by the collaboration of a group of physicians (TASAKA et al., 1967) and resulted in the emergence of the present-day gastrocamera, an instrument consisting of a lens, flash lamp, air valve and film capsule attached to a control unit by means of a 75 cm vinyl-covered tube. The tip can be deflected up or down 35 degrees to increase the field of view of the 80 degree angle of the camera lens. This instrument is passed into the stomach, which is then inflated and routine photographs taken at various depths and angles. The film may be advanced by a proximal control and 32 photographs taken in each patient in color. Since the main problems with the external camera were involved with the inability to get enough light into the stomach, and poor resolution because of the diffusion of light returning through either glass lenses or fibers, it can be easily seen that the intragastric camera did much to eliminate these factors. Excellent 5 mm pictures were obtained in color, which could be viewed with a projector immediately following development, or enlarged quite adequately for teaching or publication purposes. The instrument was fairly well tolerated by the patient with minimum preoperative medication, could be passed by physician or trained technician, and had the single drawback that all photographs taken were blind, i. e., not focussed on any particular pathology, but intended to represent all of the gastric mucosa. Ingenious methods were devised to accomplish this end, some of them rather elaborate (TANAKA, 1961; FUGIMORI, 1961; NAKAYAMA, 1964), and large numbers of gastrocameras manufactured and sold to practicing physicians in Japan, as well as to some in other parts of the world (HADLEY, 1966; LABO, 1967; MARTIN, 1967).

From the first, the advantages of the intragastric camera in producing superior color photographs of the stomach were obvious. The use of this technique as a screening method for gastric cancer, however, appeared to have some drawbacks, which will be discussed later (Chapter 2). The photographs obtained with the gastrocamera were a spur to gastroscopic photographers in general, and the combination of this camera with a fiberoptic gastroscope in 1964 appeared to be a natural and very desirable development to those who regarded gastroscopic photographs as a means of recording pathology, rather than a method of cancer screening. It became obvious that the gastrocamera-fiberscope combination visualized more lesions than the gastrocamera alone (YAMAGATA, 1963; MORRISSEY, 1966; HARA, 1967). The photographs, being directed rather than blind, were technically better. At the present, although some photographs are still taken with external cameras attached to the eyepiece of the instrument, this is necessary largely in cinegastroscopy and during biopsy, where addition of the biopsy apparatus makes inclusion of a camera at the tip impossible. The combination gastrocamera-fiberscope has become the routine gastroscopic instrument in most clinics and appears to be the most useful all-around endoscope for examination of the stomach and recording of the findings.

The fiberoptic gastroscope which served as the basis for the gastrocamera fiberscope combination, and which, like the gastrocamera, was first formally introduced in 1958, was the product of research by several individuals. The idea of transmission of light through transparent fibers was first patented in 1928 by BAIRD, but its practical application was delayed until coating of fibers was found to improve light transmission (VAN HEEL, 1954) and a practical method of fabricating fibers was discovered (HOPKINS, 1954). Following the development of a method of producing uniform-sized glass bundles by CURTISS (1957), the first fiberoptic gastroscope was manufactured in the United States, and preliminary results with this instrument were described by HIRSCHOWITZ (1961). Since then, three other manufacturers have produced instruments of this type, all of which have been modified extensively to improve their functions in different ways. The trend has been to make tips controllable, to furnish fiberoptic lighting as well as viewing, to add biopsy potential, and in some instances, to permit forward as well as lateral viewing (the standard method of most gastroscopes).

The shift from the older lens type gastroscopes of the intermediate period to the modern fiberoptic instrument has not been without trauma. The original fiberscope was highly touted as an instrument for examination of the duodenum as well as the stomach, the "gastroduodenoscope" (HIRSCHOWITZ, 1962), but other observers found that they visualized the duodenum rarely, if at all (BURNET, 1962; COHEN, 1966). The controversy engendered somewhat obscured the fact that this instrument did give excellent views of the stomach, particularly the antrum, and was more comfortable for the patient, since it was no longer necessary to hold his head stretched rigidly back during the examination. It did not operate on a fixed focus, and the angle of the lens had to be changed frequently by an adjustment near the eyepiece, a device which most found annoying. This was changed by the development of fixed-focus instruments by two different manufacturers (TSUNEOKA, 1965; KAMEYA, 1965), both of which had excellent image transmission and flexibility. No claim was made of duodenal visualization with these latter instruments. They were designed solely to examine the stomach, and were soon in wide use. One of these two, both of Japanese manufacture, was combined with the previously described gastrocamera (Olympus), and the other (Machida) was fitted with an excellent biopsy device, as well as a flash lamp and extragastric camera. A fourth fibergastroscope, of American manufacture (Eder), had forward as well as lateral viewing, and could be passed into the duodenum more readily than the other three, but has been beset with technical difficulties which are only lately resolving. With proper development, it has the potential of an excellent instrument, but early experiences have somewhat dulled its luster.

While the instruments have been experiencing growing pains, trauma of a different sort has visited the older gastroscopists. Confident in their abilities after years of experience, they suddenly (the author included) saw themselves inundated with a flood of new devices which many were loathe at first to consider any great improvement. These feelings were reinforced initially when the original fiberscope failed to live up to advance billing in visualizing the duodenum. It was also found that the new instrument, flexible as it might be throughout most of its length, had a long, rigid tip which could produce injuries, although it was originally thought to be much safer than standard gastroscopes. There was concern that inexperienced physicians might try to pass the instrument without adequate training, with the idea that it was entirely safe. The dangers were, however, properly publicized early, and emphasis placed on good training with this as with any endoscope.

It is to the credit of most of the oldsters that they were willing to change, and that all of the more active gastroscopy clinics use fiberoptics. The results produced by the instruments themselves were largely responsible for this change-about. They were demonstrably superior in revealing the stomach, recording its lesions, and recently, in delivering diagnosable pathological specimens. To be sure, there are a few instances in which the older lens gastroscopes score over the fiberscopes, and most older endoscopists keep them on hand to try out when there is an occasional failure to pass the larger diameter instrument. But for the most part, the latter is used routinely, and is here to stay. In the author's opinion, their development is the basic reason for the sudden flowering of gastroscopy in the modern period. The publicizing of these instruments and the results obtained with them should, in time, produce a considerable improvement in the diagnosis and treatment of gastric cancer, as well as the management of many other lesions native to the stomach.

Available Instruments

As a result of the rapid metamorphosis of the gastroscope during the past few years, a number of excellent instruments are available to the endoscopist. These require no particular description or listing for gastroenterologists as a whole, and those given in this section are not necessarily complete, since the technical specifications are readily available from the manufacturer. A general listing of the most useful, as well as their spheres of usefulness and special clinical qualifications, is undoubtedly in order for less interested and informed physicians, who might nevertheless wish to know their relationship to the problem of gastric cancer detection and management, and who comprise the main target for this monograph. In consideration of these readers, descriptions will be brief and to the point.

Lens Gastroscopes. As noted previously, these holdovers from the intermediate period of gastroscopy are still in use, and occasionally contribute in specific situations where the fiberoptic instrument has been tried and found wanting. Thus, where there is an inability to pass one type of instrument at the cardia or pharynx, the conventional lens gastroscope may go into the stomach, since it is of smaller diameter. Also, in some individuals, the upper body and lower fundus of the stomach may be more readily visible. The exact reason why these instruments are more successful on occasions is not always obvious, but they do have excellent viewing characteristics, and, as previously stated, at least one model has a small diameter that may be an advantage. The most advanced types, and those most widely used, are the Eder-Palmer (American manufacture) with Bernstein modification and Herman-Taylor (English manufacture). These, as well as a number of other lens instruments, are all derivations of the original Wolf-Schindler gastroscope which gave the first real impetus to gastroscopy after its invention in 1932. They may still be found in the older gastroscopist's clinics and the amount of their continued use depends to a large extent on his degree of infatuation with the fiberscope. In our clinic they have, alas, gone into almost complete eclipse.

Of the two instruments, gastroscopists in the United States are most familiar with the Eder-Palmer, which was purposely made in small diameter to pass through the Eder-Hufford esophagoscope. It has pull-wires to bend the tip downward, and excellent vision. This is the instrument which should be tried when small diameter is desired (Fig. 1). The Herman-Taylor scope is considerably larger in diameter, and has a longer rigid portion. Many British endoscopists still use this instrument.

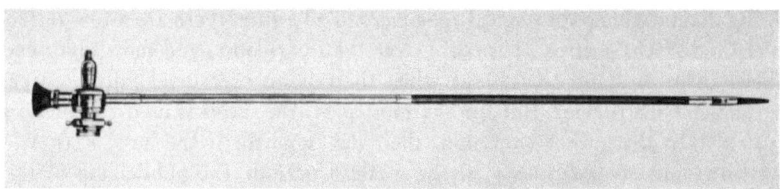

Fig. 1. Eder-Palmer gastroscope with Bernstein head modification which separates the objective slightly from the mucosa by means of a glass window. The instrument is flexible in its distal half, which may be moved in one direction by manipulation of the rachet at the head. Its small diameter and excellent lens system render it useful still when the patient has a small pharynx or cardia

Fiberoptic Gastroscopes. There are four most commonly used types of fiberoptic gastroscopes manufactured. Two are made in Japan, and two in the United States, each by different companies.

The Olympus (Japanese) fiberoptic gastroscopes come in several models, but are of two basic types, one containing the gastrocamera in the tip, and one equipped with a biopsy apparatus. Both have movable tips, may be easily passed into the antrum, and are capable of retroflexion and retrograde view. The latest model of gastrocamera fiberscope (GTF-A) is at present the best instrument for viewing and recording of the gastric mucosa, and the biopsy model (GFB) with external camera, an excellent tool for histological study. The latter model, now under development, will eventually be supplied with fiberoptic lighting as well (Figs. 2 and 3). The Olympus

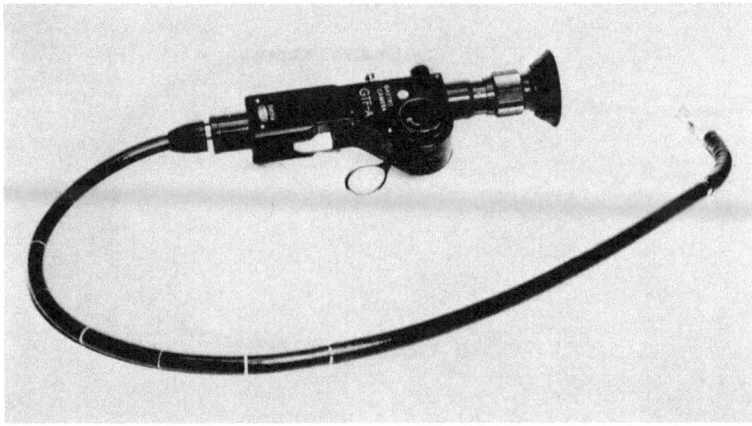

Fig. 2. Olympus GTF-A fiberscope-gastrocamera combination, showing the controllable tip feature. Thirty-two 4 mm. color photographs of excellent quality may be taken with one roll of film, which is enclosed in a tiny camera near the tip. Movement of film is accomplished by manipulation of the loop seen at the head of the instrument; the flash trigger and shutter control is just below on the instrument head. Fiberoptics of this gastroscope are superior, and all areas of the stomach may be visualized with proper positioning

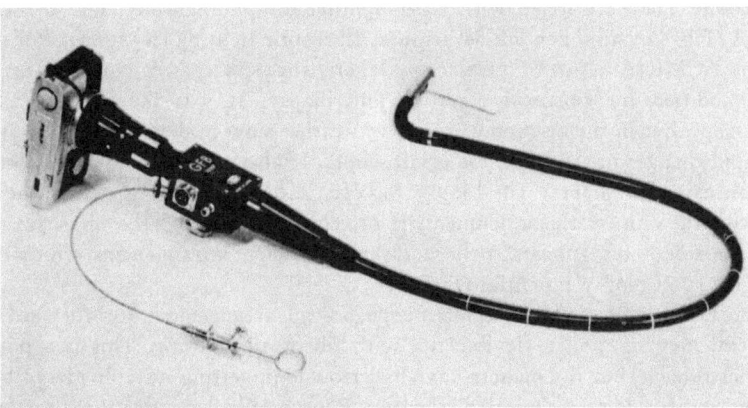

Fig. 3. Olympus GFB fiberoptic biopsy gastroscope, with external camera attached and biopsy instrument inserted (it may be seen projecting at the tip from the aperture just distal to the objective). Controllability of the tip is shown, as well as the capability of projecting the biopsy tip at right angles from the instrument. Optical system is the same as for the GTF-A, but the gastrocamera has been sacrificed for biopsy potential, and an extragastric camera is used which produces good to excellent color photographs with flash lighting

company maintains a sales and service outlet in the United States as well as several other countries, which is a distinct advantage. Gastrocamera film is developed and delivered by airmail, and gastroscopes promptly serviced.

The Machida (Japanese) instrument also comes in two basic models, the FGS-S for examination and photography with an external camera, and the FGS-B for biopsy. These are excellent instruments, although for technical reasons, photographs with the

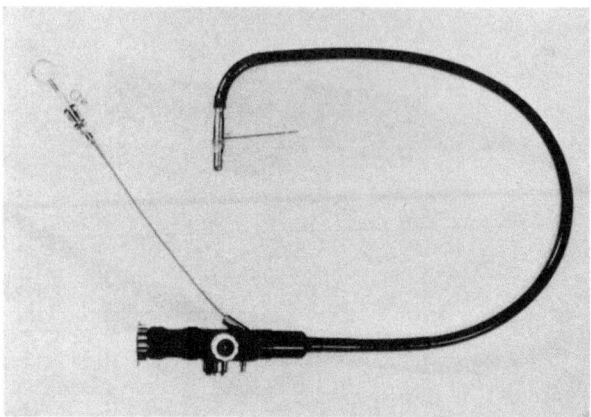

Fig. 4. Machida FGS-B fiberoptic gastroscope for examination and biopsy. Like the Olympus GFB, the tip is controllable, and the biopsy instrument inserted and manipulated in much the same fashion, although the method of raising the biopsy tip is somewhat different. Extragastric camera and flash are also available for approximately the same quality color photographs as with the GFB

internal (gastrocamera) are superior to the external camera which may be purchased to fit both. They are fitted with flash lighting for photography, like the Olympus GTF-A (Fig. 4), and a new model features fiberoptic lighting (KASUGAI, 1969).

The ACMI (American Cystoscope Makers, Inc.) fibergastroscope has been gradually modified for fiberoptic lighting and biopsy. It was the original fiberoptic gastroscope, but in the opinion of some, was rather slow in development compared to the rapid changes in the Japanese gastroscopes. It also may be used for photography with an external camera. The biopsy forceps, instead of coming out of the port in line with the axis of the instrument, is projected in front of the objective window from the side. This appears to be a rather inefficient arrangement which does not make for good biopsy potential (Fig. 5).

The Eder (American) fibergastroscope has an arrangement for forward as well as lateral viewing, and a flexible tip, with fiberoptic lighting. This is a potentially good instrument, but the makers have had trouble in getting suitable glass fibers, and it has presented some technical difficulties. Photography is with an external camera, and there is no biopsy apparatus.

The brief description of the major features of these four instruments is not intended to be complete, and details may be obtained from the manufacturers by those interested, as well as from recent reviews (MORRISSEY, 1967). The two types of instrument considered most useful for the neophyte in this field are the Olympus GTF-A for those interested in photography, and Olympus GFB or Machida FGS-B for biopsy. For those interested in good fiberoptic gastroscopes with excellent biopsy attachments, who are not purists in photography, either of the biopsy fibergastroscopes will make good all-around instruments for examination of the stomach, and rather good colored photographs can be made with the external camera with both instruments.

This section would not be complete without mention of the Olympus fiberesophagoscope, with forward viewing, controllable tip, fiberoptic lighting, and biopsy

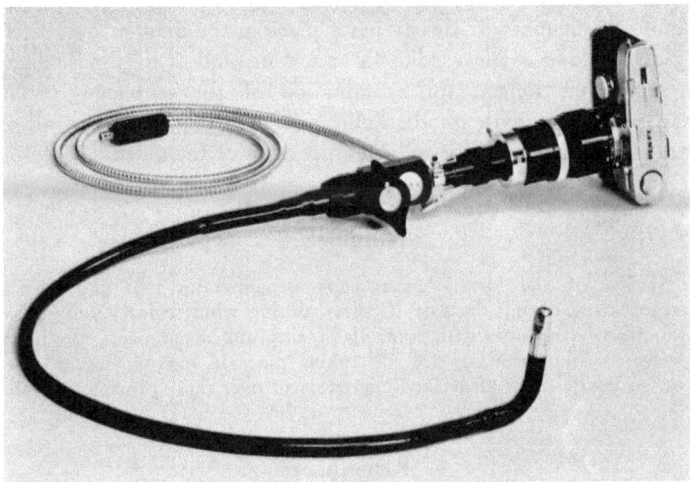

Fig. 5. ACMI Panview Mark "7" fiberoptic gastroscope with fiberoptic lighting, external camera, and biopsy potential (instrument not shown). The biopsy tip comes out of the instrument tip at the side, and has a permanent bend to bring it in view of the objective. This arrangement does not appear very efficient, although vision and maneuverability are approximately the same as with the other fiberoptic gastroscopes (Fig. 2, 3, and 4)

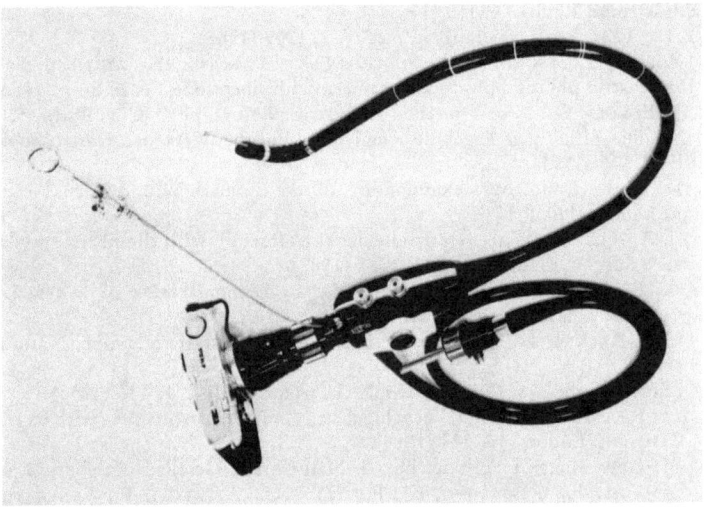

Fig. 6. Olympus EF esophagofiberscope with forward viewing, fiberoptic lighting, and apparatus for air inflation as well as fluid injection and suction cleansing of the objective. Color photographs obtained with the external camera are of excellent quality. Designed primarily for the esophagus, it is a superior instrument for visualization and biopsy of the upper half of the stomach as well

forceps (Fig. 6). Although intended initially for the esophagus, it has proven excellent for the diagnosis of carcinoma at the cardia, fundus and midportion of the stomach, as well as examination of the post-gastrectomy pouch and enterostomy openings. Photographs taken with the external camera through this instrument are unusually good, and biopsies adequate. It clearly has a place in the diagnosis of gastric cancer, particularly of the fundus and cardia. In fact, some endoscopists visualize a similar instrument, somewhat longer, for examination of the esophagus, stomach, and duodenum in succession, with photographic and biopsy potential in all three. The present instrument is too short for reliable inspection of the antrum.

Summary

A brief review of the history gastroscopy demonstrates that the most important advances have occurred during the past 10 years, during which color photography with external cameras, fibergastroscopes with controllable tips, and attachments for directed biopsy have been perfected. Improvements are still taking place in instruments and methods, but both have now reached a point of marked improvement over those previously available.

References

BURNETT, W.: An evaluation of the gastroduodenal fiberscope. Gut 3, 361 (1962).

COHEN, N. N., HUGHES, R. W., MANFREDO, H. E.: Experience with 1,000 fiber gastroscopic examinations of the stomach. Amer. J. dig. Dis. 11, 943 (1966).

CURTISS, L. E., HIRSCHOWITZ, B. I., PETERS, C. W.: A long fiberscope for internal medical examinations. (abstr.) J. Opt. Soc. Amer. 47, 117 (1957).

FUGIMORI, A.: Studies of photography of certain areas of the stomach with the gastro-camera. Gastroint. Endosc. 3, 159 (1961).

HADLEY, G. D.: The gastro-camera. Brit. med. J. 2, 1209 (1965).

HARA, Y., TOBITA, Y., TSUNODA, H., SUGIYAMA, K., ARAKAWA, F., ANSFIELD, F. J., HOON, J. R.: Intragastric photography: gastrocamera with fiberscope. Arch. Surg. 94, 337 (1967).

HEILPERN, J., PORGES, O.: A new method of gastric photography. Klin. Wschr. 9, 15 (1930).

HENNING, N.: Die bisherigen Ergebnisse und der klinische Wert der Gastroskopie. Ergebn. ges. Med. 16, 539 (1931).

HIRSCHOWITZ, B. I.: Endoscopic examination of the stomach and duodenal cap with the fiberscope. Lancet 1961 I, 1074.

— BALINT, J. A., FULTON, W. F.: Gastroduodenal endoscopy with the fiberscope—an analysis of 500 cases. Surg. Clin. N. Amer. 42, 1081 (1962).

— CURTIS, L. E., PETERS, C. W., POLLARD, H. M.: Demonstration of a new gastroscope, the "fiberscope". Gastroenterology 35, 50 (1958).

HOPKINS, H. H., KAPANY, N. S.: A flexible fiberscope using static scanning. Nature (London) 173, 39 (1954).

KAMEYA, S.: Study of the new GFS fiberscope. Gastroint. Endosc. 7, 136 (1965).

KASUGAI, K.: Recent instrumental development of fibergastroscopes with a light guide system. Gastroint. Endosc. 15, 224 (1969).

KUSSMAUL, A.: Über Magenspiegelung. Ber. d. Naturforsch. Gesellsch. Freiburg 5, 112 (1868).

LABO, G., FAGGIOLI, F., GASBARRINI, G., FONTANA, G., AZZAROLI, P., VENERATO, A.: The use of a new apparatus for gastrophotography: the gastrocamera. Arch. ital. Mal. Appar. Dig. 34, 246 (1967).

LANGE, F., MELTZING, M.: Photography of the stomach. Münch. med. Wschr. 45, 1585 (1898).

MARTINS JOB, J.: The gastrocamera. Hospital (Rio) 72, 1773 (1967).

MIKULICZ, J.: Über Gastroskopie. Wien. med. Presse 22, 1410, 1439, 1473, 1505, 1537, 1629 (1881).

MOUTIER, F.: Etude gastroscopique de l'ulcere gastrique. Presse. méd. 92, 1852 (1932).

MORRISSEY, J. F., TANAKA, Y., THORSEN, W. B.: Gastroscopy. A review of the English and Japanese literature. Gastroenterology 53, 456 (1967).

NAKAYAMA, K.: Technique of photography with Nakayama's retrograde model II gastro-camera. Gastroint. Endosc. 5, 355 (1964).

SCHINDLER, R.: Gastroscopy in thirty cases of neoplasm. Arch. intern. Med. 32, 635 (1923).

SCHINDLER, R.: La Evolucion de la gastroscopia. Med. Germano. Hisp. Am. 1, 690 (1924).
— L'Endoscopie gastrique avec le gastroscope flexible. Arch. Mal. Appar. dig. 23, 1131 (1933).
— Gastroscopy. The Endoscopic Study of Gastric Pathology. 2nd. Edition. New York: Hafner Publ. Co. 1950, p. 1.
TANAKA, Y., MORRISSEY, J. F.: An improved technique for examination of the stomach with the GT-5 gastrocamera. Gastroint. Endosc. 13, 8 (1967).
TASAKA, S., ASHIZAWA, S.: Studies on gastric diseases using the gastrocamera. Amer. Gastrosc. Soc. Bull. 5, 12 (1958).
— SAKITA, T.: Progress of gastrocamera examination. Proceedings of the First Congress of the International Society of Endoscopy. Part 2, 70 (1967).
TSUNEOKA, K.: A description of Japanese (Machida) fiberscope. Gastroint. Endosc. 7, 134 (1965).
UJI, T.: The gastrocamera. Tokyo Med. J. 61, 135 (1952).
VAN HEEL, A. C. S.: A new method of transporting optical images without aberration. Nature (London) 173, 39 (1954).
WALK, L.: The history of gastroscopy. Clin. Med. 1, 209 (1966).
YAMAGATA, K., MIURA, K., OSHIBA, S., VENO, K., KIKUCHI, R.: Experience with a fiberscope. Gastroint. Endosc. 5, 104 (1963).

Chapter 2

Endoscopic Methods in Cancer Diagnosis

Routine Examination

Traditionally, the routine screening examination for gastric cancer in symptomatic or asymptomatic individuals has been roentgenoscopy, rather than endoscopy. Even intubation gastric analysis is usually considered a traumatic procedure, although it may prove useful in determining a certain group of potential victims. Insertion of a larger instrument for routine surveys is probably out of the question in the United States. Radiological screening of the general population has not been very productive, although in selected groups (GILBERTSON, 1967) a certain number of cancers may be discovered.

In addition, the decreasing incidence of gastric cancer in the U.S., as well as the heterogeneity of the population, and the widespread practice of private, rather than socialized medicine, make it difficult to establish any screening program for this purpose. At the present time, surveys of this type will undoubtedly be of small groups, and, if successful, have little effect on the mortality of gastric cancer as a whole.

Japan, on the other hand, with a very high incidence of gastric cancer and a more systematized type of medical practice, has been able to perform surveys for cancer on hundreds of thousands of individuals, employing both routine x-ray examination and gastrocamera photography as the initial screening devices. The reported results, while probably not applicable to other countries except perhaps Iceland, Finland, or Chile with similarly high incidences of gastric cancer do give an indication of the value of such surveys, of which endoscopy (gastrocamera and fibergastroscope studies) is an essential part.

Radiological and Gastrocamera Survey

The standard survey endoscope is the Olympus GT-5A gastrocamera, which, although it does not allow one to inspect the mucosa under direct vision, usually gives adequate views through the medium of colored photographs taken with the stomach inflated and the instrument rotated into various routine positions. The instrument has been in widespread use for roughly 10 years, and a late report states that a total of 15,801 gastrocameras are now used clinically in Japan (KASUGAI, 1969). There are also numerous centers where physicians are trained in gastrocamera photography and the interpretation of photographs.

The initial survey, which may be made of symptomatic or asymptomatic individuals, also comprises roentgenoscopy with a number of routine views recorded on film, gastric analysis and stool examination. Suspicious findings are further investigated by more sophisticated x-ray evaluation, fiberoptic gastroscopy, gastric washing for cytology (often under direct vision through the gastroscope), and gastric biopsy where indicated. A minimum of sedation or anesthesia is used during these procedures, which are presented as routines.

A recent report by ARIGA (1967), describes the Japanese methods of survey and results which are representative of their experience. The study begins with personal interviews and photofluorography, which screens out all but 20 per cent. These individuals are then subjected to endoscopy, routine x-rays (with double contrast techniques if indicated), and cytology. The end result is approximately 10 per cent of the original group, who exhibit cancer, polyp, ulcer, or other pathology. In Japan in 1964, a total of 210,017 persons were examined, 0.26% of whom were found to have gastric cancer. In 1965, 333,531 were examined and gastric cancer discovered in 0.27%, a remarkably consistent figure. During this period there were in Japan 155 clinics and doctors' offices where such mass surveys were conducted, consisting of 23 university hospitals, 81 other hospitals and 51 public and civil offices. This is a tremendous effort, which can only be admired. Even more significant is the number of patients found who had gastric cancer confined to the mucosa or submucosa, with corresponding improvement in operability and prognosis. A report by YAMAGATA (1967) gives these figures as 4.8% in 1955 und 1956, 10.8% in 1959, 15.9% in 1964, and 34.5% in 1966. The Japanese workers attribute this steady improvement in early cancer diagnosis to their advanced methods of screening of large numbers of individuals. A further study by NAKAYAMA (1969) is also optimistic as to the use of surveys in asymptomatic patients in Japan.

From the endoscopic point of view, however, it is difficult even for the enthusiast to determine exactly what the contribution of endoscopy, either the simple gastrocamera or the more sophisticated gastrocamera-fiberscope, has been in this effort; however, one report by KUROYANAGI (1968) is fairly informative. Comparative reports are available (HARA et al., 1966; MORRISSEY, 1968) which appear to show that the gastrocamera is probably not as efficient as the gastrocamera-fiberscope in diagnosing gastric cancer. Presumably, the two methods, endoscopy and roentgenoscopy, complement each other when used together in the examination of large numbers of individuals. However, the method of survey as described by ARIGA appears to show that x-ray is the only definitive means of diagnosis employed on the first screening, which reduces the total number being evaluated by 80%. It would be interesting to see what results might emerge if both x-ray and gastrocamera were used in the initial screen, difficult as this might become. This difficulty is emphasized by a survey of 300 Japanese subjects who had undergone gastrocamera examination, of whom 60 per cent said they had subsequent discomfort, and 30 per cent stated they did not wish a repeat examination (TAKEZOE, 1964).

Thus, while it may be taken for granted that endoscopy of the stomach has made a significant contribution to the diagnosis of gastric cancer in large numbers of individual patients, its value as a screening procedure is still unclear. What is evident, and emphatically so, is the contribution the Japanese have made in clarifying many aspects of the disease, improving all features of available endoscopes, and demonstrating what can be done with them. A more precise analysis of the endoscopic contribution in Japan over a longer period of time will undoubtedly give an answer to the question of its true contribution in screening surveys. The employment of the more advanced gastroscopic techniques and instruments, in which the Japanese have been leaders, has universally valuable and practical applications to gastric cancer everywhere, even in countries like the United States, where the incidence of this type of neoplasia is decreasing.

Endoscopic Evaluation of Symptomatic Individuals

The major employment of gastroscopy for the diagnosis of gastric cancer in most countries is in the symptomatic patient who has usually had a roentgenological examination prior to being seen by the endoscopist. The idea has become firmly fixed in many quarters that x-ray examination is a superior method for discovering gastric cancer which seldom fails. As a result, the endoscopist is usually concerned with those patients in whom the radiologist has been unable to make a firm diagnosis, or who have some major contraindication to surgical exploration in the face of a suspicious x-ray finding. He is, consequently, at a disadvantage from the start. It is most discouraging to be confronted, as often happens, with a patient who has had several inconclusive roentgenological examinations over a period of months, with persistent symptoms, and to find on gastroscopy a large lesion which in all probability could have been recognized and biopsied months earlier. This is not to belittle the value of x-ray examination, which does indeed discover most gastric cancers. It is, however, a method with failings like all others, and the physician is too often lulled into a false sense of security by a negative examination. The plea is only that x-ray and endoscopy ideally complement each other, one frequently giving information that the other cannot.

This concept has become well established in cancer of the rectum, where everyone agrees that the barium enema should always be followed within a couple of days by a sigmoidoscopy, or vice versa, but somehow there is a great deal of resistance to adopting routine endoscopy of the esophagus and stomach. There are readily discernible, if no longer valid, reasons for such an attitute. Esophagoscopy and gastroscopy are still regarded by some as operative procedures (and performed in operating rooms, complete with surgical gowns!). Actually, with the presently available instruments which have been developed within the past 10 years, both procedures are well on a par with sigmoidoscopy, and so performed by most gastroenterologists, in a treatment room with a minimum of bother and disturbance to the patient. The accidents which plagued the older endoscopists still occur, as they do with any instrumentation, but they are rare, and becoming rarer, as the new and the old generations alike learn to use the very flexible fiberscopes (MORRISSEY, 1967; KATZ, 1969). The stomach can now be viewed in its entirety, all interesting features recorded in color, and (one insuperable advantage impossible with x-ray) the gastric mucosa may be accurately biopsied at will. There is no present way in which one may ascertain how many gastric cancers could be discovered at an early stage if routine endoscopy were added to x-ray examination. The Japanese studies indicate that the endoscopic contribution might be considerable. Likewise, our experience makes us believe that many useless laparotomies, undertaken on the basis of inconclusive x-ray findings, sometimes in bad risk patients, might be avoided by endoscopy. There are good reasons, therefore, why endoscopy of the stomach should be used in a more routine manner if gastric cancer is suspected. These are largely the employment of a technique which in recent years has been markedly improved in accuracy, safety and acceptability, and the evidence that it can give information prior to surgery which is often impossible to obtain by any other method.

At The University of Texas M. D. Anderson Hospital and Tumor Institute, gastroscopy has been routinely employed in the diagnosis of gastric lesions with or without positive x-ray findings where the clinical situation appeared to warrant such routine use. Unfortunately, most of the patients referred to a cancer institute have advanced disease, or have already been explored and found inoperable. It has become evident that routine endoscopy at this level will not change the mortality from gastric cancer, but may be of great value in the management of the individual patient. To reach its true potential, however limited, gastroscopy must be employed either personally or through a consultant by the patient's personal physician. This objective will take years of education of the physician and the training of many more endoscopists than are presently available. Perhaps an advance may be realized through the regional center program in the United States, but so far no organized attempt has been made. The potential is there, however, and although endoscopy is unsuitable for survey use in the United States and most other countries, routine gastroscopic study will eventually prove extremely valuable in the diagnosis and management of gastric cancer.

Gastroscopic Photography

Attempts to record gastric lesions during endoscopy gave unsatisfactory results for many years, despite the fact that the value of photography was early recognized. The first intragastric cameras were essentially unsatisfactory, and it was not until TASAKA and ASHIZAWA (1958) presented some excellent colored photographs obtained with the GT-5 gastrocamera at the World Congress of Gastroenterology in Washington, D. C. that the intragastric camera was seriously considered in gastric photography. Their instrument had been under development since 1950. Many attempts had also been made to take colored photographs with extragastric cameras attached to the eyepiece of lens gastroscopes, with varying degrees of success. Fair to good results had been obtained with large tungsten lamps by SEGAL and WATSON (1948) and NELSON (1956), but it was not until electronic flash lighting was employed by DEBRAY and HOUSSET (1958), that really excellent color photographs were taken through the lens gastroscope with the external camera.

The first fiberscope was also presented at the 1958 World Congress and it appeared certain that color photography would materially advance through the medium of this new type of endoscopy. As most gastroscopists have gradually turned to the fiberoptic instruments, photography has rapidly improved from tungsten light sources through the electronic flash to fiberoptic lighting, which is gradually becoming routine with all new models. The latter has the advantage of carrying light from external sources into the stomach, leaving the tip of the instrument cool (the large tungsten lamps heated badly and sometimes produced burns) and permitting almost unlimited illumination. Resolution was poor with early fiberglass bundles, but this factor has been markedly improved, and since fiberglass will transmit 2.5 times as much light as glass lenses, it is easy to see why present fiberscopes so equipped are producing excellent still and cine photography (COLCHER, 1967).

Gastric color photography since 1958 has been in a steady state of flux. Most pioneers with the external cameras were overjoyed with the improvement from the old tungsten lighting to electronic flash and lens gastroscopes (NELSON, 1960, 1962). The fiberscope-gastrocamera combination was then produced and tried, and it became obvious that this instrument, with electronic flash, produced photographs with the best resolution and acceptable color, as well as having the advantage of visualizing many more areas of the stomach than the lens gastroscope could negotiate. The majority, who were satisfied with still photographs, were perfectly willing to settle down with this instrument for the long haul (OTAKI, 1969; PERSYKO, 1969). Then another advance unsettled this situation, and again opened the question of the external camera. This was the addition of the guided biopsy instrument to the fiberoptic gastroscope.

It has always been true that just so much can be added to an instrument which must go through the cardia and be manipulated in the stomach. The biopsy apparatus, when added to a fiberscope, evicted the gastrocamera. The endoscopist who wishes to biopsy the stomach with present instruments must either pass the gastrocamera-fiberscope first and take his pictures, or be satisfied with photographs obtained with the external camera attached to the eyepiece. Pictures taken with these latter instruments equipped with electronic flash lighting have been acceptable, but hardly equal in resolution to the gastrocamera photographs. With the addition of fiberoptic lighting, however, photographs are being produced with the external cameras which are almost as good in every way. Those obtained with the new fiberoptic esophagoscope, which may be passed into the upper stomach and is equipped with forward viewing as well as a means of thoroughly cleaning the objective, are truly excellent. They no doubt have provided the inspiration for the addition of fiberoptic lighting to the new model Olympus GFB, which is to be available in 1970, and may well resolve the dilemma of gastric biopsy and photography with the same instrument in one passage.

The purpose of gastroscopic photography has been in some contention. Originally developed primarily with external cameras, it was conceived with the idea of recording pathology for study and demonstration. With the advent of the very successful GT-5 gastrocamera, blind photography was advocated for the discovery and diagnosis of gastric lesions, independent of true endoscopy. The Japanese have unquestionably demonstrated that this can be done, but since the majority of opinion appears to be that the fiberscope-gastrocamera combination is more efficient (HARA, 1966; MORRISSEY, 1968), there is some question as to whether this type of employment is justified, especially in the United States or other countries with a low incidence of gastric cancer. Our experience has been that reliance on blind photography may produce errors which can be eliminated by combining photography with thorough endoscopic examination (NELSON, 1966). In the latter procedure, photographs are used to record characteristics of the individual lesions for future study and teaching purposes. The ability to biopsy most gastric lesions has also altered the whole concept of endoscopy, and gastroscopists now wish to document their visual impressions with histologic proof obtained on the initial examination. Experience shows that no matter how well trained the physician, observation alone can go only so far, and isolated photographs may, in particular, be deceiving. At present it seems best to advise that the entire stomach be evaluated by fibergastroscopy, any lesions recorded in color for future demonstration, and biopsied if at all possible.

Cinegastroscopy has likewise been advocated as a means of determining the malignant nature of a lesion, because disturbed peristalsis, easily demonstrated by this method, may signify malignant infiltration (COLCHER, 1967). Unfortunately, while it is certainly true that extensive malignant neoplasia interferes with peristalsis, the same effect may be seen with long-standing and extensive inflammatory change, somewhat vitiating this criterion. Likewise, localized malignancies may interfere very little with peristalsis, and there is the final limiting factor that during gastroscopy, peristalsis is seldom observed outside of the antrum. Therefore, while cinegastroscopy is very worthwhile for teaching purposes, it probably has little place in the routine photography of patients (MORRISSEY, 1967).

Before leaving the general discussion of photography, a few words on technique are appropriate, since it may be assumed that some readers are ardent endoscopists. Those who came into gastroscopic photography the hard way, during the early years of experimentation, learned that the basic rules apply in the stomach just as they do elsewhere. The camera records only what it sees, and if its vision is obscured by blood or mucus on the objective, if the angle of vision is tangential, or if there is too much motion, poor photographs will result. Gastric photography has become so simple with the gastrocamera as to somewhat obscure these facts, and as a result many of the pictures displayed at meetings are only fair quality. They usually show recognizable lesions, but often poorly, when a little care with the cleaning of the objective, framing of the picture, and having the patient hold his breath would produce infinitely better results. These maneuvers were always necessary with the early, crude apparatus (NELSON, 1966), and they still make the difference between passable and superior photographs.

Whatever the method used, the development of reliable gastric color photography has been a major step in the advancement of gastroscopy. Skepticism has been somewhat dissipated, the particular characteristics of many types of pathology much better delineated and understood, and teaching advanced immeasurably. Color photography has given the gastroscopist a medium in which to exhibit his findings, and even those who never look through a gastroscope can appreciate how accurate these findings have become. The method can well be said to have paved the way for the next, and probably final development, that of guided biopsy under direct vision.

Gastroscopic Biopsy

SCHINDLER, although recognizing the value of biopsy, doubted the possibility of obtaining adequate specimens. He did, however, experiment with an early model of KENAMORE (1940, 1946), attached to the outside of the standard gastroscope, although the results were poor. A later model by BENEDICT (1948) featured a forceps which was passed through the shaft of the instrument, and then raised into view with a small elevator. This was a bulky instrument, and more often than not, only the shaft of the biopsy forceps was visible to the operator. There was no control of the gastroscope tip, and while some good biopsies were obtained, results in general were so discouraging that the instrument was to a large extent abandoned. Other more recent models featured suction as well as forceps instruments, but were also too inefficient for reliable results (TOMENIUS, 1952; BERRY, 1961; DEBRAY, 1962).

The most recent instruments, made by the Olympus and Machida manufacturing companies of Japan, employ two principles which have made directed gastroscopic biopsy practical. In both, the biopsy forceps is passed through the shaft of a fiberoptic gastroscope, but instead of emerging proximal to the objective, a main defect of the Benedict apparatus, they present distally, and are then elevated back into view so the tip, and not the shaft, is clearly visible. The second improvement is development of a controllable gastroscope tip which may be moved in two directions, providing another means of angling the biopsy forceps. Both of these instruments have been used extensively in Japan, and are presently being evaluated elsewhere. Positive biopsies were obtained in 126 of 154 proven gastric cancers by KASUGAI (1966), and 88 per cent of 113 cancers by HAYASKI and SUGIURA (1966) with the Machida FGS-B, while positive biopsies were taken in 90 per cent of gastric cancers by TOBITA and HARA (1967) with the Olympus GFB fiberscope.

Lesions as small as 2 mm. may at times be biopsied with these gastroscopes, although it should be noted that those most experienced in their use admit that the upper body, cardia and distal antrum are difficult areas, and such pinpoint accuracy is not to be expected in these locations. It is also recommended (KASUGAI, 1966) that 4 to 8 biopsies be taken from each lesion or suspicious area. From these observations and the reported accuracy, it may be seen that gastroscopic biopsy is still not a simple procedure unattended with frustration.

Our experiences with one of these instruments over the past year have borne out both the good and bad points enumerated by the original workers. We found that guided biopsies could be taken by experienced endoscopists with relative ease and surprisingly little practice. The tissue obtained is often insufficient for diagnoses of diffuse lesions such as gastritis because of the shallow bite of the biopsy tip, designed for safety rather than complete sampling, and possessed of no cutting edge. The tissue is grasped and torn off by traction, not incision. We confirmed the fact that even when a malignant process appears grossly extensive, multiple biopsies should be obtained or the procedure may have to be repeated. In several instances, however, repeat attempts have been successful in diagnosing carcinoma, and led to the hope that more experience will reduce the necessity of multiple attempts to a minium. It is humbling and salutary to find that one's visual acumen may not be quite as unfailing as had been thought, when the forceps grasps, under direct vision, what is obviously tumor but which turns out to be benign inflammatory tissue.

We were also able to confirm the fact that the upper third of the stomach and distal antrum are more difficult to biopsy than the remainder. However, persistence led to several triumphs in these areas, and the upper stomach should be vulnerable to biopsy with the fiberoptic esophagoscope, although our experience with this instrument has been limited. In addition to the location of lesions, other simple factors such as the inability of the patient to retain air for one reason or another, excessive secretion of mucus or regurgitation through the pylorus during the necessarily prolonged procedure, bleeding following the initial biopsies or inability to pass the relatively large tip of the instrument through the cardia in massively involved stomachs, were all limiting factors. Japanese workers report that early cancerous lesions are biopsied with greater accuracy than more diffuse carcinomas. This may appear paradoxical unless it is realized that small lesions disturb the stomach as a whole very little. Inflation is good, with correspondingly good visability and maneuverability. This principle undoubtedly holds for all gastric lesions: the smaller the pathology, the less the disturbance of gastric visability, and the better the opportunity for biopsy.

The most obvious improvement which should be made in this apparatus is in the biopsy forceps head. The instrument itself is surprisingly rugged, considering its length, and unusually maneuverable. What is needed is a cutting tip, which would have to be little or no larger than the present one, but would allow reasonable amounts of tumor to be excised, rather than torn, off. It would be necessary to use such a cutting head with great caution in biopsying normal mucosa, but even here it might have value in selected instances. The present rather weak cupping arrangement seldom gets near the muscularis, in our experience, and usually slips off any hard, smooth tumor surface. A recent model features a central pin between the cups, on which the tumor surface may be impaled. This device is successful in a limited degree only, since while it does help to fix the tissue, it fragments the small biopsy. The excellent sections of tissue, demonstrated in Japanese publications, apparently produced by use of these instruments have, in our experience, not been approached (SHIRAKABE, 1966).

Despite these limitations, the present instruments must be considered a great advance. An 80 to 90 per cent accuracy in diagnosing gastric cancer is not to be disregarded, and our preliminary trials would indicate that these figures are no exaggeration. In all likelihood, however, the Japanese see and biopsy many more early malignant lesions than will be available to their conterparts in the United States and most other areas, a fact that should be understood in comparing results. The smaller lesions are obviously more amenable to biopsy.

Another useful feature of the biopsy fiberscopes which should be mentioned is the ability to selectively wash, under pressure, localized areas of the mucosa and collect the washings for cytologic study. An accuracy of 96.8 per cent in diagnosing cancer by this method has been reported by KASUGAI (1969). It seems that this would be particularly applicable in inaccessible areas such as the antrum, where results have been poor with standard lavage. The washing is accomplished by passing a plastic tube through the biopsy channel, which directs the stream to the selected site. The gastroscope is then removed, a gastric tube inserted, and the aspirate processed in the usual manner. We have not attempted this maneuver, but it would appear especially useful in cases where direct mucosal biopsy was negative but the gross examination remained highly suspicious.

Summary

Endoscopy plays a definite, although not too well-evaluated a part in screening cancer surveys in Japan, which have resulted in the diagnosis of an appreciable number of cases of early gastric cancer. Such surveys are probably not practical in other countries, where the initial finding of cancer is usually by roentgenoscopy, and endoscopy figures mainly in evaluation of such findings. More routine use in all areas, however, would probably result in earlier diagnosis and therapy, particularly since modern gastroscopes represent a considerable improvement over older instruments, and offer the advantages of direct viewing of the lesion, color photography, and biopsy. These features of gastric endoscopy, so far meagerly exploited, represent real advances in the management of gastric cancer if properly employed.

2*

References

ARIGA, K.: Statistics of gastric cancer found by gastric mass survey in Japan. Nihon Univ. J. Med. **9**, 175 (1967).

BENEDICT, E. B.: An operating gastroscope. Gastroenterology **11**, 281 (1948).

BERRY, L. H.: Direct vision suction gastro-biopsy assembly: demonstration (presented before annual meeting of Amer. Gastroscopic Society, Cook County Hospital, Chicago, May, 1961).

COLCHER, H.: Cinegastroscopy with two new gastroscopes. Amer. J. Gastroent. **47**, 16 (1967).

DEBRAY, C., HOUSSET, P.: Color gastro-photography with electronic flash. Amer. Gastrosc. Soc. Bull. **5**, 9 (1958).

— — MARTIN, E., BOURDAIS, J. P., NICOLAIDIS, C. L.: A new direct-vision biopsy gastro-scope. Gut **3**, 273 (1962).

GILBERTSON, V. A., WANGENSTEEN, O. H.: Gastric analysis as a screening measure for cancer of the stomach. Cancer **20**, 127 (1967).

HARA, Y., TOBITA, Y., WATANABE, M.: Clinical use of gastrocamera with fiberscope (GTF) for detection of gastric and hepatic pathologies. Proceedings of the First Congress of the International Society of Endoscopy. Tokyo (Japan): Hitachi Printing Co. 1966, p. 206.

HAYASHI, K., SUGIURA, Y.: Direct biopsy and abrasive cytology with the $FGSB_3$ and B_4 (Machida). Gastroint. Endosc. **8**, 37 (1966).

KASUGAI, T.: Study of direct washing cytology and direct biopsy with the fiberscope for gastric cancer. Gastroint. Endosc. **8**, 48 (1966).

— Endoscopy in Japan with special reference to detection of gastric cancer. Gastroint. Endosc. **15**, 204 (1969).

KATZ, D.: Morbidity and mortality in standard and flexible gastrointestinal endoscopy. Gastroint. Endosc. **15**, 134 (1969).

KENAMORE, B.: A biopsy forceps for the flexible gastroscope. Amer. J. dig. Dis. **7**, 539 (1940).

— SCHEFF, H., WOMACK, N. A.: Study of gastric lesions by means of biopsy specimens removed endoscopically. Arch. Surg. **52**, 50 (1946).

MORRISSEY, J. F., TANAKA, Y., THORSEN, W. B.: Gastroscopy: a review of the English and Japanese literature. Gastroenterology **53**, 456 (1967).

— — — The relative value of the Olympus model GT-5 gastrocamera and Olympus model GT-F gastrocamera fiberscope. Gastroint. Endosc. **14**, 197 (1968).

NAKAYAMA, K.: Gastric cancer: the success of early detection by a coordinated program of periodic gastric mucosal x-ray studies and gastroscopic and gastric camera observations. Surgery **65**, 227 (1969).

NELSON, R. S.: Intragastric photography. Amer. J. Gastroent. **45**, 255 (1966).

— A comparison of electronic flash and tungsten light gastroscopic color photography. In: Current Gastroenterology. New York (N. Y.): Paul B. Hoeber Comp. 1962, p. 47.

— Gastroscopic Photography. Chicago (Ill.): Year Book Med. Publ. 1966.

— Routine gastroscopic photography with an electronic flash. Amer. Gastroc. Soc. Bull. **5**, 9 (1958).

OTAKI, A. T., DUNDAS , T., GILL, A. M.: Experience with the fiberscope-gastrocamera. Amer. J. Gastroent. **51**, 187 (1969).

PERSYKO, L., SWIFT, J. E., VENKATACHAIAM, B., SEREBRO, H. A., BECK, I. T.: Diagnosis of pathological changes in the stomach by gastroscopy Still and cine colour photography using a new fiberoptic gastroscope. Canad. med. Ass. J. **100**, 1067 (1969).

SEGAL, H. L., WATSON, J. S., JR.: Color photography through the flexible gastroscope. Gastroenterology **10**, 575 (1948).

SHIRAKABE, H., ICHIKAWA, H., KUMAKURA, K., NISHIZAWA, M., HIGURASHI, K., HAYAKAWA, H., MURAKAMI T.: Atlas of X-ray Diagnosis of Early Gastric Cancer. Philadelphia (Pa.): J. B. Lippincott Co. 1966.

TAKEZOE, K.: The problems of endoscopy. The ability and practice of the gastrocamera on the mass medical examination. Abstracts of papers presented at the sixth annual meeting of Japan Gastroenterological Endoscopy Society, April (1964).

Tobita, Y., Hara, Y.: Studies on the gastric biopsy and brushing by gastrofiberscope with angle-change (Olympus GFB). Proceedings of the First Congress of the International Society of Endoscopy, p. 328 (1967).

Tomenius, J.: A new Instrument for gastric biopsies under visual control. Gastroenterology 21, 544 (1952).

Yamagata, S.: Epidemiology and Symptomatology of Early Cancer of Stomach. In: Recent Advances of Gastroenterology, Vol. 1. Proceedings of the Third World Congress of Gastroenterology. Tokyo (Japan): Nonkodo Co. 1967, pp. 487.

Chapter 3

Specific Pathological Conditions Related to Gastric Cancer: Gastroscopic Diagnosis in Benign and Malignant Disease

The diagnosis of gastric cancer is often made more difficult and confusing because of the gross resemblance of other pathological and clinical entities to malignant neoplasia. These similarities, noted both on roentgenoscopy and on inspection of the resected specimen, may be so great as to render certain lesions indistinguishable, benign from malignant, or vice versa. The experienced surgeon, long plagued by diagnostic errors, both of omission and commission by radiologists and clinicians, may be forgiven, to some extent at least, his tendency to explore in any equivocal situation.

It has become apparent, however, to ourselves as well as to many others that gastroscopy frequently has a great deal to offer in resolving these dilemmas. Indeed, the time may well have been reached when an accuracy of 95 to 98 per cent can be expected if the patient is expertly examined by the combination of roentgenoscopy and gastroscopy (plus biopsy) alone. Documentation of this belief is extremely difficult because of the infrequent use of endoscopy in diagnosis, even in some of the older and more revered institutions of medicine. In addition, most of the few available studies showing the value of the combined approach were carried out using the older gastroscopic instruments, and the results are hardly valid today. Standard texts are replete with descriptions of the diagnosis and treatment of gastric lesions which contain little information on gastroscopy, and fewer recommendations for its use (CECIL, 1959; HARRISON, 1962). Those brave souls who would at least like to mention gastroscopy favorably seem to have a tendency to overemphasize its complications and shortcomings (MONAGHAN, 1963; OLSEN, 1964). These are real enough, but should be considered in context, in the same manner that the risks of surgery must be taken into account when this method is advocated for all suspicious lesions. Endoscopy of the stomach today can be undertaken in almost all poor surgical risks with considerable equanimity, and the same cannot be said for surgical exploration. If even a few of these patients can be spared the risk of surgery by a much lower-risk procedure, it is our position that it should be carried out. The advantages, physically and economically, in the good risk group are also obvious.

In light of the fact that insufficient studies are available to determine the exact value of gastroscopy in gastric cancer, and considering the rapid advances which have been made in instrumentation in the past 10 years (which have not yet been assimilated), it is difficult to make a precise statement as to the usefulness of gastroscopy in the various confusing benign conditions which have come to be associated with gastric cancer. Certain information from previous studies, however, as well as preliminary observations over the most recent years, allow an approximation of the status of this method in diagnosis and evaluation. Some of the following remarks may be, therefore, more in the realm of predictions than positive statements, which is probably all that is possible at present in this rapidly changing scene. If endoscopists are right in their projections, instrumentations will completely alter the diagnostic aspects of gastric cancer within the next few years. In no field will this change be more profound than in the confusing conditions of ulcer, polyps, and gastritis, as well as in carcinoma and lymphoma.

Gastric Ulcer

Ulcers of the stomach, large or small, seem to present one of the major problems in cancer diagnosis. This appears to be so baffling to some as to elicit such statements as that of STOUT (1967), "The chief reason for the still high death rate from gastric cancer seems to be the insidious development of many cases and the difficulty of making an early differentiation between simple ulcer and cancerous ulcer. It is beyond the scope of this preface to enter into the debate concerning this subject which has been raging for at least 25 years. The writer will only state that if, at his present age, it should be demonstrated that he had an ulcer of the stomach, he would want an immediate operation without any period of waiting to find out whether or not it was cancerous." This statement from the foreword of an outstanding and recent text on neoplasms of the stomach (McNEER et al., 1967) seems to adequately express the conclusions drawn later in the section on "Small Gastric Ulcerations." According to these published figures, x-ray was correct in 53.5 per cent of benign, and 23.0 per cent of malignant ulcers, incorrect in 17.6 of benign, and 37.0 per cent of malignant ulcers, with inconclusive findings in 26.4 and 40.0 per cent of benign and malignant lesions, respectively. Gastroscopy fared worse; it was incorrect in 30.1 per cent, correct in 30.1, and inconclusive in 39.8 per cent of benign ulcers, while findings were correct in only 25.0 per cent, incorrect in 41.7 per cent, and inconclusive in 33.3 per cent of malignant ulcers. In another section of the same volume, however, accuracy of roentgenology and gastroscopy used together to detect cancer is given as 96.4 per cent. It appears, therefore, that malignant ulcers are being placed in some special category. Certainly, they cannot be included in the figures for gastric cancer; the overall inaccuracy would be much greater.

Gastric ulcer seems to occupy some special niche, a high point of invulnerability to diagnosis, in the minds of these and other authors. Some of the statistics (McNEER, 1967), however, are difficult to understand. How could radiologists and gastroscopists have been allowed so much leeway in diagnosis as to give "inconclusive" readings in such a high incidence of benign and malignant ulcers? Surely if one is expert, he should be required to give his opinion, for good or ill, based on his demonstration of the lesion in more cases than this. Were they unable to demonstrate the ulcer to their satisfaction? Or merely unable to make up their minds? No answer is forthcoming, but the discrepancy seems disproportionate, and casts some doubt on the whole study. In addition, the number studied (144 patients) appears entirely inadequate for the institution involved, and the instruments employed, outmoded.

In contrast, there are other published papers in which both roentgenoscopy and gastroscopy were used to diagnose gastric ulceration with somewhat different results. SCHINDLER and DESNEUX (1953) found that 239 of 273 gastric ulcers were diagnosed correctly (48 malignant, 191 benign), while 20 were incorrectly diagnosed, 18 rated malignant being benign, and 2 called benign being malignant. Fourteen were inconclusively classified, of which 9 were benign and 5 malignant. DODD and NELSON (1961) reviewed 100 consecutive gastric ulcers, evaluated by both x-ray and gastroscopy, and found an overall accuracy of 95 per cent. Thirteen ulcers (mostly of the lesser curvature of the antrum) were not visualized with the older semi-flexible gastroscope, which did, however, show 8 ulcerations not seen on x-ray examination. Colored photographs were used to demonstrate gastroscopic criteria for benignancy or malignancy, and these as well as the roentgenologic criteria held up well in evaluation.

In the more modern era of the fiberscope and gastrocamera, endoscopic observations have been carried out on the appearance and course of healing of gastric ulcers over weeks and months (SAKITA et al., 1967; Ariga et al., 1967), with careful classification as to the gross types and their healing characteristics. These were all correctly diagnosed by x-ray and gastroscopy. COHEN et al. (1966) also reported 90 per cent accuracy in evaluating malignant gastric ulcers with the fiberscope.

In our own experience, a great deal of confidence has developed in our ability to differentiate between benign and malignant ulcers, whatever their size. Those still confused about gastric ulcer seem to be the ones who have made no real trial of endoscopy, or, indeed, much else besides roentgenoscopy and observation. Many of them apparently are unaware of the fact that color photographs may be made of almost all gastric ulcers for classification of gross features, and very few seem to have heard of directed gastric biopsy in diagnosis.

A large number of gastric ulcers have been seen and studied on the gastroenterological service of the M. D. Anderson Hospital and Tumor Institute, both in- and out-patient. Careful evaluation of each lesion by roentgenoscopy, gastroscopy with color photography, and for the past year, directed biopsy has resulted in a very high degree of accuracy. Although there may be an occasional equivocal diagnosis endoscopically, we are beginning to believe that virtually all of these may be eliminated by the use of directed biopsy, and now use it routinely in such instances. Excellent follow-up is available in almost all patients, and so far as can be ascertained, very few cancerous ulcers have been misdiagnosed during the past 12 years. Our main endoscopic error has been over-diagnosis, in that a few very large ulcers have been incorrectly diagnosed as malignant, only to prove benign on resection. In general, although no statistics have been gathered, accuracy is at least as good as that noted in a previous publication (DODD and NELSON, 1961), and probably somewhat better since the use of fiberoptic gastroscopy and gastrocamera. A more recent prospective study of the factors in healing and recurrence of gastric ulcers was carried out in 16 veterans administration hospitals, using only radiological criteria for diagnosis and follow-up. Of 638 patients, the ulcer was classified as radiographically "apparently benign" in 574, and "indeterminate" in 64 (11.1%). During a 2 year follow-up, surgery was advised in 102 patients. Cancer was found in 3.3 per cent of the "apparently benign" ulcers and 9.4 per cent of the "indeterminate" group. The incidence was 10 per cent in ulcers larger than 300 mm² (product of width times depth), and 2.2 per cent in the smaller ones. It would appear that even when roentgenoscopy alone is used in evaluation, risk from cancer in the small gastric ulcer is exceedingly low, and indiscriminate resection unjustified. If gastroscopy had been added to the study, even better results could have been expected, especially with guided biopsy.

So far as our personal experience is concerned the "small gastric ulcer" is less difficult to diagnose than the large, deep ulcer with heavily indurated margins. The smaller lesions are easier to expose and examine endoscopically, and follow-up gastroscopy is also much simpler. We believe that the differential between benign and malignant ulcers is not particularly difficult in these patients, but that it is important to resect those which fail to heal because of the life-threatening complications which any such ulcer may present, even though it is benign. In all but a few patients, the malignant ulcer may now be diagnosed immediately, and referred for resection without an expensive and time-consuming waiting period. Furthermore, since a fair number of ulcers are found only by gastroscopy, no examination is complete without the use of this method.

Gastroscopic Criteria. The majority of gastric ulcers may be correctly diagnosed on their gross characteristics alone. These have to do with the form of the crater and the surrounding mucosa. The sharply demarcated or "punched-out" crater, intact in all quadrants, in a smooth and uninfiltrated surrounding area, is unequivocally benign (Figs. 7, 8, 9, 9a, 10 and 11). The floor is usually covered with mucus, and if there has been recent bleeding it is evidenced by a clot filling the crater, or several blackish areas in the mucus denoting small bleeding points (Figs. 12 and 13). Converging folds are less frequently seen at gastroscopy than at roentgenoscopy, since air insufflation tends to iron them out, but when present they run to the edge of the ulcer. Alternatively, the crater floor may be covered with necrotic debris. In acute benign disease, the surrounding mucosa usually exhibits marked inflammatory change, which on follow-up visualization will be seen to have disappeared (Figs. 14 and 15). All ulcers should be followed to complete healing gastroscopically, since with treatment they may disappear radiologically long before they have healed gastroscopically.

The malignant ulcer in the majority of patients we see appears from the beginning as ulcerating tumor, rather than ulcer alone (Figs. 16 and 17). This is apparently not so true of Japan, where a fair number of early lesions present largely as ulcer, with minimal surrounding carcinomatous infiltration. Massive or minimal, the carcinomatous infiltration appears as fixed nodules, folds, or tumor mass. The lesion is often slightly raised above the surrounding area, and the Japanese describe a "step-down" edge to the ulcer crater which they feel is pathognomonic of malignancy. Even in Japan, where the screening process discovers so many more early lesions than are seen in the United States, endoscopists feel quite confident in their ability to diagnose an ulcer on gross characteristics, and to follow it in safety where conservative therapy seems indicated. UTSUMI et al. (1967) followed 95 patients with ulcers by gastrocamera photography for intervals ranging from 3 years to 9 years and 3 months. All were judged benign at the beginning of the study, and none became malignant, although various characteristics appeared to be factors in the individual healing process. SATO and WADA (1967) reported on their serial fibergastroscopic observations in 43 patients, of whom 6 were "ulcer-carcinoma", and the rest benign.

They attached great importance to the irregularity of the ulcer wall and margin as well as "irregular prominence" of the ulcer bed. Complete recovery was noted in more than 80 per cent in 3 months if the ulcer margin was sharp and crater smooth. SAKITA et al., (1967) followed 302 gastric ulcers, of which 57 were "early stage of gastric cancer with ulceration." Only 7 of the latter showed any major change; this consisted in necrosis of the ulcer edge. There was no tendency for healing, which was exhibited to a greater or lesser degree in all of the benign ulcers. Our experience has been similar, in that the few malignant ulcers we have followed have never shown any evidence of healing (NELSON, 1966).

The small minority of ulcers which fall into the indeterminate group because of confusing characteristics are of two types. The first, by far the more numerous, is the large, chronic-appearing ulceration with marked infiltration around the edges. Despite the infiltration, the edge of the ulceration may be entirely clear and sharp. In our experience, the majority of this type of ulcer, all of which have been resected because of possible malignant degeneration, have been benign (Figs. 18 and 19). The differential here is not in the crater, but in the infiltration, and may be impossible grossly. Before the advent of guided biopsy, there appeared to be no possible way to determining the nature of such ulcers. Now, through the medium of multiple biopsies of the infiltrated edge, an immediate differential may be made in most patients.

Case Report. A 49-year-old white female was seen in consultation for gastroscopy only which was carried out on two occasions. A marked inflammatory reaction was noted with a lesser curvature ulcer crater at the apex of converging folds (Fig. 18). A biopsy was taken which revealed nonspecific chronic gastritis (Fig. 18 a). X-ray findings were completely indeterminate as to the nature of the lesion. The patient underwent resection with the findings of benign gastric ulcer with marked chronic inflammatory infiltrate.

Case Report. This 83-year-old white female had been ill for two years with post prandial epigastric pain. There was occasional vomiting which had become so severe that she had lost a total of 22 pounds and had become quite anorexic with evidence of overnight food retention. Gastroscopy on June 17, 1968 showed benign gastric ulceration involving the immediate prepyloric region on the anterior wall and lesser curvature, with evidence of considerable chronic inflammation. She also was found to have uncontrolled diabetes mellitus. Following treatment for her diabetes and her ulcer she improved considerably. Because of the chronic nature of the ulceration, surgery was offered but was refused by the patient. In February 13, 1969 the ulcer was again visualized and there appeared to be little change (Fig. 19). Biopsies were taken at this time which were essentially unremarkable, showing no evidence of tumor or ulceration. When last seen, approximately 14 months after her initial examination, gastroscopy showed no real change in the lesion and the general condition of the patient was good.

The second type of ulcer with non-diagnostic gross features is small, the edge is fairly sharp, and the infiltration at the edge may be minimal or confusing, consisting of slight elevation of the mucosa around the crater (Fig. 20), or fixed radiating folds which appear to almost, but not quite, lead into the ulcer crater (Fig. 21). This latter type causes considerable concern since it represents the most difficult malignant lesion to diagnose endoscopically. In our experience it is extremely rare; in a 12 year period, 4 of this type were discovered among gastric ulcers seen at The University of Texas M. D. Anderson Hospital. None have been found since the advent of biopsy, but it is possible that the small directed biopsy instrument would not have been of much help, since in 2 patients diligent search of the permanent pathologic sections of the gross specimen was necessary to detect early malignant change. We assume that this is really the feared "small gastric ulceration." If so, we can only state that they are rare but do not heal, and therefore come eventually to surgery in any well-conducted endoscopic follow-up clinic.

Gastric Biopsy. The advent of the guided biopsy instrument inevitably led to speculations that routine biopsy of the questionable ulcer would solve the problem of diagnosis. We have felt, however, that the real test would come in biopsying all visualized gastric ulcers routinely and comparing the results with those found on follow-up either by complete healing over a period of time under endoscopic observation, or surgical resection. We have initiated such a study, which is still in the preliminary stages. However, in the first 19 ulcers, the accuracy of biopsy has been 94 per cent. Seventeen of these lesions were benign. Another, which fell into the first type of the indeterminate group mentioned above massively infiltrated at the edges, showed unequivocal carcinoma in directed biopsies of the raised area at the edge of the crater. The final lesion, a shallow ulceration which did not heal, was found on resection to be a superficially ulcerating carcinoma. The edges of the ulcer showed no tumor, but a raised area in the crater was positive. This bit of observation has been tucked away for future reference, since it would appear to mean that "islands" of tissue seen in ulcer craters should always be biopsied, as well as the periphery.

The criticism can, and undoubtedly will, be raised that a negative biopsy will not rule out carcinoma. While perfectly correct, it overlooks the fact that the biopsy diagnosis of ulcers is largely confirmatory of the gross appearance at the initial examination and follow-up. Observation of hundreds of ulcers over extended periods of time has been necessary to convince us that a correct diagnosis may be made with roentgenoscopy and endoscopy alone. The application of directed biopsy in an additional large number of lesions will be necessary to determine its exact role. The preliminary opinion would be that it will be very useful in resolving the occasional equivocal case, but that in most instances it will render only complementary information to the gross appearance of the ulcer. This type of study should be carried out on a large scale in numerous institutions, since it is certainly true that many of the carcinomatous lesions referred to a cancer institute are well-established, though ulcerating, tumors, and the value of biopsy should be ascertained in all types of patient populations, preferably those of large general hospitals.

The Japanese, who have had the most prolonged and extensive experience in diagnosing early gastric cancer, apparently do not attempt to make any real differentiation as to whether the lesion is ulcerating or non-ulcerating. They do not seem to fear the "small gastric ulceration", but subject all suspicious areas of the stomach to exhaustive examination, and certainly their success in discovering early cancers is considerably better than other published results. KASUGAI (1969) reporting from the Aichi Cancer Center Hospital in Nagoya, Japan, where 10 endoscopists examine 60 to 80 cases a day, 3 days a week, reports the following results in gastric cancer; diagnostic accuracy by endoscopy was 95.1 per cent (early gastric cancer 98.1 per cent, advanced gastric cancer 94.6 per cent), diagnostic accuracy of gastric lavage cytology under direct vision was 96.8 per cent (early gastric cancer 96.9 per cent, advanced gastric cancer 96.4 per cent), diagnostic accuracy of gastric biopsy under direct vision was 87.6 per cent (early gastric cancer 92.3 per cent, advanced gastric cancer 86.6 per cent), and diagnostic accuracy of x-ray examination was 90.0 per cent (early gastric cancer 84.0 per cent, advanced gastric cancer 95.0 per cent).

These results are impressive and certainly worth investigating in large scale studies in the United States and elsewhere, even though the survey methods which originally brought the patients to this cancer center may not be practicable. They should give pause to those who would submit all patients with a roentgenologic diagnosis of gastric ulcer to early exploration and resection. There is an appreciable primary mortality from gastric resection, particularly in the cancer age group which may, with our newer methods of diagnosis, well be prohibitive if a blanket policy of surgery is advised. To put it bluntly, the unreasonable fear of the "small gastric ulceration" may produce more deaths than cancer of the stomach, and quite unnecessarily. We believe that present methods of diagnosis, particularly those advanced by the Japanese and only recently being investigated in other areas, make such a policy obsolete. It will probably be a long time before there is general agreement on this point, but matters have already progressed far enough so that no physician can afford to approach the question of gastric ulceration in such a superficial manner as to send all ulcer patients to surgery.

Gastritis and Gastropathies

Gastritis is in general a controversial subject, one to which gastroscopy has perhaps lent as much confusion in the past, based on gross observations, as it is now lending light through the medium of guided biopsy. Many of the gross observations of the earlier endoscopists have been discredited through biopsy, and have had to be unlearned in order to clarify thinking on gastritis. Much confusion and many unanswered questions still remain which are not germane to the subject at hand, i. e., endoscopy in gastric cancer. There is no doubt that cancer is found more frequently in stomachs diffusely involved with atrophic gastritis and gastric atrophy, but in many cases, this is not the background, and the mucosa surrounding a cancer may be essentially normal histologically, with adequate secretion of acid from the stomach. Although earlier workers felt that cancer largely developed on a background of gastritis (KONJEZTNY, 1938) modern students of this subject feel that the old, involved classifications of gastritis are unjustified (SCHINDLER, 1947), and that while cancer may occur in association with a damaged mucosa, the relationship is obscure (STOUT, 1953).

Our main concern is the confusion that may be caused in diagnosis between chronic gastritis, gastropathies, and cancer on a morphological basis by roentgenoscopy and gastroscopy. In our experience, there are two main types of involvement which may cause confusion: 1) chronic inflammation of the antrum, and 2) the "gastropathy" of giant hypertrophy of the gastric mucosa (Menetrier's disease). Both of these conditions at times produce diagnostic dilemmas although more often to the roentgenologist than the gastroscopist.

Antral Gastritis. Inflammatory changes in the antral mucosa, which differs histologically from that of the rest of the stomach, are a common accompaniment of antral ulceration. During the acute phase, there may be marked edema and distortion of folds (Fig. 22), which may disappear completely, or develop into a chronic phase with scarring, roughening, and repeated periods of ulceration (Fig. 23). The end process of such chronic inflammatory change may well be loss of distensibility, some interference with peristalsis, and actual cicatricial deformity of antrum, pylorus, or both (Fig. 24).

We have observed several such patients over a period of months, and it appears obvious, on comparing accuracy of diagnosis by roentgenoscopy and gastroscopy, that the former is no match for the latter, if performed with the modern fiberscope, gastrocamera, and directed biopsy, since such an antrum frequently has all the x-ray characteristics of early or late malignant disease. Many of these patients do eventually come to surgery because of the high degree of obstruction that may ensue over a period of time. Thus far, we have found the endoscopic procedures accurate in predicting the histological diagnosis, and feel that there is a definite advantage in proper presurgical evaluation, particularly in the elderly (most prone in our experience to develop the chronic lesion), and those with contraindications to surgery. It should be admitted that we feel much safer in following such patients medically since biopsy has become available, but have also been happier with our greater degree of latitude in those who might well not survive resection. Other types of gastritis, which do not deform the antrum, are detected only by gastroscopy (Fig. 25). Incidentally, it should be stated unequivocally since the opposite opinion has been expressed so many times, that biopsy within the antrum with the fiberoptic biopsy instruments is now quite simple in the majority of patients, and multiple samplings may be taken with safety.

It is our definite conclusion that all roentgenologically deformed antrums should be investigated gastroscopically. Cancer appears in the antrum more frequently than in any other part of the stomach, and abnormalities in this area are consequently more suspect. In many older or debilitated patients the proper evaluation of such deformities may be of vital importance. With gastroscopy and biopsy, the diagnosis of antral cancer is usually simple. That of chronic antral gastritis is more difficult, but quite feasible. There is no other method, short of surgical exploration, which will allow a firm opinion.

Giant Hypertrophy of the Gastric Mucosa (Menetrier's Disease). Various degrees of "hyperrugosity" are frequently observed radiographically, and may be quite puzzling at times to the radiologist, who lacks the ability to distend the stomach maximally with his barium medium. In most such cases, definite conclusions can be drawn by the gastroscopist, who can usually inject enough air to compress normal or edematous gastric folds in all areas of the stomach. When folds are prominent, stiff, and fail to flatten out at endoscopy, it may be presumed that pathology is present, although the exact diagnosis of gastritis, hypertrophy, carcinoma or lymphoma must be established histologically.

Diffuse thickening of the gastric wall by excessive proliferation of the mucosa, first described by MENETRIER (1888), is a relatively rare entity, but occurs often enough to cause problems, particularly in a cancer hospital, which is the recipient of many out-of-the-way radiologic abnormalities. The roentgenologic appearance frequently simulates carcinoma or lymphoma. The mucosa is massively hypertrophic, and may be covered by thick mucus when viewed gastroscopically, or appear to have small superimposed polypoid excrescences on top of the folds (Fig. 26). Most of the cases described in the literature involve large areas of the stomach, particularly the greater curvature (MATZNER et al., 1951; MORAN, 1959; FIEBER, 1955), but the disease may be localized, and one of our patients with histologically proven disease exhibited only two polypoid folds, grossly diagnosed as adenomatous polyps (NELSON, 1966), prior to resection. Another (NELSON, 1954) underwent total gastric resection at an early age because his stomach cavity was so full of hypertrophied, polypoid mucosa, and the wall so stiff, that he could no longer eat without pain and distention. Most patients' disease falls somewhere between these two extremes. The other characteristic described by Menetrier in one of the patients contained in his original report is that of protein loss, which is now quite well accepted, based on the results of several studies (BALFOUR et al., 1950; CHARLES et al., 1963; CITRIN et al., 1957), to be the result of loss through the hypertrophic gastric mucosa. While edema and hypoproteinemia, plus hypertrophied gastric folds should always be considered Menetrier's until proven otherwise, hypoproteinemia is not necessarily a part of the histological entity of the disease, and it is the abnormal folds, after all, which produce confusion with neoplasia (Fig. 26). None of our six histologically proven cases (two only reported) had protein loss, yet in all patients carcinoma was considered because of the gross appearance of the mucosa by roentgenography, gastroscopy, or both. In three other patients with typical gross findings only, one had low serum proteins of undetermined etiology, but unfortunately refused further evaluation.

Many patients with Menetrier's disease have minimal symptoms, and are understandably reluctant to undergo extensive studies or surgery based on the rather vague explanation which the physician may have to offer. The problem in judgement is further compounded by the fact that carcinoma has been observed in conjunction with hypertrophic gastropathy in a small number of patients, some of whom have had histologic confirmation of their disease. The difficulty of evaluating such reports was well shown, however, by TEXTER et al. in their 1953 study. They were able to gather five previously reported patients, only one of whom, on searching review, appeared valid. Their own single patient, who was followed to postmortem examination, obviously developed carcinoma while under observation for proven Menetrier's. Subsequent reports over the years continue to show this association (GAMES et al., 1966; CHUSID et al., 1964). Opinion appears to be divided as to whether hypertrophic gastropathy is truly a precursor of carcinoma. Some observers (SPELLBERG et al., 1953; KENNEY et al., 1954) seem to feel that such progression is a strong possibility, if not a probability. In a recent pathological review, BUTZ (1960) notes that although STOUT (1943) found an increase of the mucin-producing cells and felt that this might be a metaplasia preceding carcinoma, there is no evidence that carcinoma follows this transformation. None of the 14 patients he studied had developed cancer.

Regardless of whether Menetrier's disease is or is not a pre-neoplastic lesion, two points are worthy of note from a practical standpoint. The first is that the differential from neoplasia may be impossible on gross observation by any means, and that adequate biopsies must therefore be obtained in all questionable cases. The second is that in a number of cases in which carcinoma has developed, the patient has been under observation with a diagnosis of hypertrophic gastritis or gastropathy for a number of years before cancer apparently occurred—how many is undetermined, since neoplastic changes may well be masked by Menetrier's.

Gastroscopy has been well recognized by most as an excellent diagnostic adjunct to roentgenology in this disease (SPELLBERG et al., 1953; MAIMON et al., 1947), and at least one observer has expressed the hope that gastroscopic color photography might help in its recognition (KENNEY et al., 1954). It can be stated that such pictures do help (NELSON, 1966) in demonstrating gross features and in follow-up. In one of such instances, a patient was followed over a four-year period, during which she was

photographed first with the older method of electronic flash through the lens gastroscope, and finally twice with the gastrocamera-fiberscope (Fig. 27). In this case, follow-up photography had the advantage of demonstrating progression of the process
from the antrum to involvement of the greater curvature. Mainly, however, photographs serve as training aids, and certainly must be supplemented with adequate
biopsy. The case report on this patient with changing gastroscopic features is presented below.

Case Report. A 67-year-old white female was first seen February 20, 1964 because of
stomach pains and roentgenograms reported to show a tumor of the stomach. Gastroscopic
examination one week later revealed many large hyperplastic-looking folds with nodules on
the surface. There was no evidence of ulceration or tumor formation and antral peristalsis
was normal. This was felt to be Menetrier's disease. A repeat examination six weeks later
gave the same findings and the same diagnosis. Since she had had evidence of gastrointestinal
bleeding in the past and was still having pain, it was felt that she should have subtotal
gastric resection. Biopsy was taken at surgery but no resection was carried out because frozen
section revealed no tumor. Further study of the biopsy resulted in revised findings and a
diagnosis of Menetrier's disease. The patient has been followed since 1964 with repeat gastroscopic examinations and the only complication noted has been an iron deficiency anemia
which responded to oral iron therapy. On the last gastroscopic examination on July 10, 1969
more than five years after her original study, large folds could still be seen in the antrum
but now the involvement seemed to be more extensive with spread to the greater curvature
side of the stomach. There appeared to be no reason to change the diagnosis and no evidence
of carcinoma was noted. She remains on follow-up.

There is some question as to whether the small biopsy instruments now available
for the fiberscope are adequate to diagnose Menetrier's. In the only patient with
grossly typical folds and hypoproteinemia which we have had the opportunity to
biopsy with this equipment, it was possible to see some signs of inflammatory change,
but the specimens were not adequate for positive identification. They appear to be
too superficial, and are frequently small in size. This is therefore one area in which
guided biopsy at gastroscopy is inadequate at the present time. Larger biopsy tips
may solve the problem in the future, but while gastroscopic biopsy should probably
be tried when the patient exhibits typical features, open biopsy may well be necessary
for a firm diagnosis in Menetrier's disease. Having established the diagnosis, follow-
up in the uncomplicated case which does not require surgery is better carried out by
endoscopy documented by color photography, biopsy, and gastric cytology where indicated than by roentgenoscopy.

Adenomas and Benign Polypoid Tumors

Adenomas. Adenomatous polyps of the stomach are relatively rare, and due to
the paucity of symptoms associated with these tumors, it is probable that many are
never detected during the lifetime of individuals harboring them. When they do
produce symptoms, however, or are accidentally discovered during the course of
roentgenoscopy or gastroscopy performed routinely in the evaluation of some gastrointestinal complaint, they present a problem that requires careful solution, since a
certain number are malignant rather than benign. Just how high this number is, and
whether many benign adenomas undergo malignant degeneration, are questions which
may be argued interminably. The simplest solution, and one urged by all surgeons, is

to remove such lesions when found. Statistics would support this reasoning in the majority of patients because of the excellent results obtained following the resection of malignant polyps. This simplistic approach cannot be uncritically accepted, however, because in the age group in which most adenomatous polyps are found, degenerative and other diseases often present a distinct threat during any type of major surgery, and some of such patients may refuse surgery. Unfortunately, most of the optimistic reports of results on surgery for adenomas fail to mention the routine complications and operative deaths which must, nevertheless, be taken into account by the truly thoughtful physician.

Presented with the dilemma of the roentgenologically discovered polyp in a patient who is obviously a poor risk by reason of cardiac, pulmonary, renal or other contraindications, what can the gastroscopist do to help resolve the question of which is the greater risk, the resection, or the polyp? Most texts consign gastroscopy to a minor role in this and other situations involving polypoid lesions of the stomach (McNeer and Pack, 1967; ReMine et al., 1964). Our experience has been otherwise. Roentgenograms do very well when they demonstrate the single tumor, if this is all that is present. Modern gastroscopy even here may contribute materially by producing colored photographs of such lesions taken from different angles which are more definitive in every way than roentgenograms (Nelson, 1966). When multiple adenomas are present, roentgenoscopy in our experience has usually given a completely inadequate picture of the true situation, which has been corrected in convincing fashion by gastroscopy and photography. It is not unknown, in fact, for even the surgeon to have extreme difficulty in finding small gastroscopically-demonstrated adenomatous polyps at the time of gastrotomy. This has happened several times on our service.

Most endoscopists, therefore, have difficulty in understanding the attitude that endoscopy is without value in polyposis (McNeer and Pack, 1967). A complete evaluation of the gross picture in polyposis of the stomach is usually possible by no other means preoperatively. This is obviously not the whole story, however, and a second question must be asked: can the malignant or benign nature of a polypoid lesion be determined unequivocally preoperatively by gastroscopy? The honest answer at present must be: in most cases, no (Palmer, 1949, 1965).

The ability to thoroughly visualize gastric polyps, and accurately estimate their location and shape, should not, however, be underestimated. As an example, it is interesting to note the various sizes of tumors in series where roentgenograms have been used almost exclusively to evaluate the question of polyps. In one recent publication (McNeer and Pack, 1967), over half the lesions (27) were 3 cm or greater in diameter, and 17 were 6 to 11 cm. The trained gastroscopist may be pardoned if he questions the classification of lesions of this size, poorly visualized by x-ray examination, as possible benign polyps. Many of them, gastroscopically speaking, would obviously fall into the classification of polypoid cancer from the start, like those shown in Figs. 32 and 37, where there was no question in the mind of the endoscopist that the findings represented cancer.

It seems that a thorough study should be made of patients with polypoid lesions, employing the most modern techniques of both roentgenoscopy and gastroscopy, before a real decision can be made as to the relative values of the two methods in evaluating these tumors. At present there is no justification for statements that

gastroscopy is useless or less effective than roentgenoscopy, and where these senti-
ments are expressed a strong suspicion must be entertained that endoscopic methods
either have been employed infrequently, or inadequately by poorly-trained personnel
or those unfamiliar with the more modern techniques.

Our experience would indicate that the smaller adenomatous polyps are much
better delineated by gastroscopy than any other means (GARRY, 1959; DI BIANCO et al.,
1965), particularly when multiple, that carcinomatous infiltrations in association with
benign polyps are better seen, and may presently be biopsied to provide a definite
diagnosis in the same manner as other carcinomas. This latter aspect has been quite
important, since very few of the polyps we have seen in the stomach have appeared
to be undergoing malignant degeneration, and carcinoma, when it has appeared with
polyps, has in all but two patients been a separate and gastroscopically recognizable
lesion. This is, of course, if one disregards the large polypoid carcinomas which seem
to have been included under adenomatous polyps in some series.

An example of the latter point is the patient whose gastroscopic photographs are
shown in Figs. 28 and 29.

Case Report. This 84-year-old white male was seen for gastroscopy because of epigastric
pain and routine x-ray which had shown polyposis of the stomach. He also had a history
of heart disease and probable emphysema. Polyps were noted, involving the floor of the
antrum, lesser curvature and one area which appeared to be infiltrated submucosally.
Another large polyp was noted on the posterior wall and another in the fundus on a broad
base. Biopsies were taken which showed adenocarcinoma (Figs. 28a and 28b). The patient
was referred to his physician for treatment. He refused surgery, and was placed on 5-
Fluorouracil. Four months after his initial examination he had gained several pounds and
was asymptomatic. Repeat gastroscopy showed little change in his lesions, and no growth of
carcinoma.

Our experience has led us to speculate as to whether the more important relationship in polyposis and cancer is not whether a polyp may become malignant, but
whether the type of background mucosa seen in both these diseases is not more likely
to develop both cancer and polyps, for reasons which are at present unclear. At any
rate, we have learned to carefully search all areas of the stomach involved with
polyps, especially when they are multiple. Authorities agree that cancer is more likely
to develop in stomachs with multiple, as opposed to single polyps, and that has been
our experience as well. In fact, we have yet to find a singly-occurring polypoid lesion
which was cancerous from the gastroscopic standpoint, providing always that the
large, obvious polypoid carcinomas are excluded from this classification, as mentioned previously.

Case Report. A 64-year-old white woman had complaints of epigastric and right quadrant pain coming on in attacks for at least 10 years, sometimes associated with nausea and
vomiting. She was referred with a diagnosis of cancer of the stomach, on the basis of roentgenograms which showed a poorly defined mass in the stomach. Repeat roentgenological
studies revealed a benign-looking gastric polyp, as well as cholelithiasis. Gastroscopy confirmed the diagnosis of benign polyp, shown in Fig. 30. Cholecystectomy and resection of
the polyp were successfully carried out, both diagnoses being confirmed histologically. She
was asymptomatic when seen as an outpatient 18 months later.

Comment: The original x-ray was interpreted as carcinoma because of poor technique. This was corrected by a better study and gastroscopy plus color photography,
but is typical of many x-rays submitted to our institution, which are of poor quality

and would lead to substantial error without improved roentgenographic technique and gastroscopy.

It must appear to the reader by now that we feel that gastroscopy is a more reliable means of determining the malignancy of the individual polypoid lesion than roentgenoscopy. This is true. Our experience, confirmed by clinical correlation, is that most polypoid lesions have been correctly diagnosed by gastroscopy in terms of gross characteristics supported by photographic representation.

Directed gastroscopic biopsy of benign polyps, as opposed to biopsy of polypoid carcinoma, has, however, in our limited experience proven disappointing. It is perfectly possible to seize even the small .5 cm. diameter polyps with forceps, but to date the biopsies obtained have shown only normal mucosa, despite repeated attempts, in three patients. This appears to be due to the very small size of the forceps provided, although KASUGAI (1969) reports the removal of a benign polyp with the Machida biopsy gastroscope. Obviously, the ability to biopsy polyps at intervals might be a key point in the follow-up of aged or poor-risk individuals with single benign-appearing polyps, but the available instruments leave doubt that they can be relied upon for this purpose at the present time. An improved instrument with cutting head probably would solve this problem, and development of such a biopsy forceps should be a prime concern of the manufacturers.

The gastroscopist, like the radiologist, must freely admit that while almost all polyps have been correctly evaluated it is impossible to differentiate with absolute certainty between benign and malignant polyps on gross characteristics alone without biopsy. Biopsy is obviously impossible during roentgenoscopy, but can be performed during gastroscopy. The larger polypoid lesions of the stomach, which are almost all malignant, may be easily biopsied at gastroscopy, with a high degree of accuracy. The smaller polyps, almost all benign, nevertheless exist in a type of mucosa which may at some future date produce carcinoma, if it is not present at the initial study. Small polyps are difficult to biopsy adequately. These being the facts, it appears that all questionable polypoid lesions should be removed when there is no serious contraindication to surgery. As noted previously, polyps tend to occur in an age group where such contraindications are common. If this is the situation, negative gross and microscopic gastroscopic findings may be acceptable indications and conditions for long-term follow-up without surgery. We have several such patients on routine outpatient status with interval evaluation at present, with no indication of the development of cancer. Others have reported similar experiences (PAUL and LOGAN, 1947; YARNIS et al., 1952; CAREY and HAY, 1948). As a final note, it appears that all patients with roentgenologically-demonstrated polypoid lesions should be gastroscoped. In a number of cases these findings have been demonstrated gastroscopically to have been caused by bezoars or other foreign bodies (Fig. 55) (NELSON, 1963).

Other Benign Polypoid Tumors. All members of this group are rare, but all have been visualized endoscopically. The most common appears to be heterotopic pancreas, which in our experience has always appeared as a submucosal, smooth, and obviously benign tumor. We have found more of these gastroscopically on our service than have been demonstrated radiographically (NELSON, 1958).

Others include hamartomas (NELSON, 1959), lipomas (most rare), and leiomyomas. The latter is best evaluated gastroscopically because of its tendency to ulcerate and present the radiographic picture of benign ulcer in some patients. Tumors of this type are always obvious tumors at endoscopy, and the ulceration can be clearly seen to be part of a submucosal mass. Unfortunately, no distinction can be made gastroscopically between leiomyoma and leiomyosarcoma (NELSON, 1968).

Carcinoma

There is at present every indication that gastroscopy is seldom employed in the diagnosis of carcinoma of the stomach in the United States. MORRISSEY et al., in a recent comprehensive review (1967) report statistics from the Japanese literature only, a sad commentary on its use in this country, and an excellent documentation of its aggressive employment in an area where the incidence of gastric carcinoma is approximately four times that in America. In a recent study conducted in seven hospitals scattered throughout the United States (5), Canada (1), and Hawaii (1), only 23 per cent of 1241 gastric cancer patients were gastroscoped. Individual hospitals varied from 3 to 69 per cent, the latter figure coming from the M. D. Anderson Hospital and Tumor Institute, where endoscopy is apparently more routinely carried out than in other institutions.

It is at present impossible to estimate the exact contribution which gastroscopy might make in the management of gastric cancer. Most cases can be readily diagnosed and treated on the basis of roentgenograms, but it is surprising how much may be added to the evaluation of the individual case by endoscopy. This may take the form of confirmation of the diagnosis of cancer in a radiographically suspicious lesion, differentiation of carcinoma from lymphoma, delineation of the gross involvement, occasionally visualization of a cancer unsuspected radiologically, or the reversal of a firm radiological diagnosis of cancer. As has been emphasized several times previously, newer instruments and techniques within the past few years have made most standard texts on this subject obsolete. Gastroscopy will in most cases allow the physician to proceed on the firm grounds of objective findings where previously there were many unanswered questions.

Primary Carcinoma. Once again it appears necessary to reiterate that it is now gastroscopically possible to visualize the antrum and fundus completely with the newer instruments, since textbooks still describe these as partial "blind areas." Even with the older lens gastroscopes, lesions of these areas could be seen and photographed in some patients (NELSON, 1966). A good example of what may be seen in the fundus by retroflexing the fibergastroscope is shown in Fig. 31. The case report follows.

Case Report. A 49-year-old white male who had been under treatment for tumor of the retromolar angle, squamous cell type, was referred because of epigastric distress, and roentgenograms of the stomach had shown a highly suspicious lesion of the fundus with narrowing of the esophagogastric junction. A repeat x-ray examination revealed a lesion which was unequivocally diagnosed as carcinoma of the fundus of the stomach. Tumor nodules were noted in the gastric fundus with some reduction in overall volume. At gastroscopy nothing was seen in the antrum or body but on the retroflex view there was a nodular infiltration on the posterior wall of the fundus which grossly had the appearance of carcinoma. This area was biopsied twice but showed only a moderate infiltrate of plasma cells. No tumor was found. Surgery was carried out ten days later and there was evidence of marked chronic inflammation and fibrosis involving the liver and posterior wall of the fundus of the stomach. Biopsy showed nonspecific granulomatous inflammation in the lymph nodes which resembled sarcoid although this diagnosis could not definitely be made histologically. Seven months later the patient on follow-up therapy to his mandible, was asymptomatic as regards his stomach.

Comment: The nodular appearance of this lesion was suspicious for cancer gastroscopically, but the biopsies were negative. The x-ray diagnosis was unequivocally cancer. At this stage of its development, directed biopsy probably cannot be relied upon entirely unless a positive diagnosis of some kind can be made. Expertise and confidence in this technique have both increased since this patient was studied.

The body of the stomach is usually visualized equally well by both roentgenoscopy and gastroscopy. However, the clarity of the endoscopic picture by gastroscopy is not appreciated by most physicians. Thus, the radiographically indistinctly seen "polypoid mass" shown in Fig. 32 is obviously a fungating polypoid carcinoma to the gastroscopist. The ulcers shown in Figs. 33, 33a, 33b, 34 and 35 are definite ulcerating carcinomas. The constricted gastric lumen of the patient represented by Fig. 36 was highly suspicious of carcinoma by both x-ray and gastroscopy, but it remained for the newer technique of guided biopsy to confirm the diagnosis, as described in the following case report:

Case Report. This 45-year-old Latin American male complained of abdominal pain radiating around to the midback. He had a history of gastrointestinal hemorrhages beginning three years previously, and been diagnosed as having peptic ulcer. Roentgenograms revealed a probable neoplasm in the stomach with associated epigastric mass. There appeared to be extensive submucosal infiltration with severe distortion of the normal mucosal pattern. Peristalsis remained however, and the stomach showed a reasonable degree of distensibility. On gastroscopic examination, it was difficult for the patient to hold air and all folds looked heavy and edematous but no true evidence of tumor, inflammation or ulceration could be made out. Although suspicious, it was impossible to make a gross diagnosis of carcinoma. Two biopsies were taken which revealed mucin-producing adenocarcinoma (Figs. 36a and 36b). The patient elected to be treated in Mexico and was lost to follow-up.

The diagnosis of carcinoma of the antrum is relatively simple in most patients. The carcinoma may partly block the antrum, as in Fig. 37, but the nature of the disease is plain and biopsy confirmatory. In the more distal antrum, represented by Fig. 38, the deformity produced by cancer of the pylorus is quite obvious. The superficially spreading carcinoma (Fig. 39), with shallow ulceration, is somewhat more difficult, but again the area is stiff, peristalsis goes through the remainder of the antrum normally, and directed biopsy confirms the visual impression.

Recurrent Carcinoma. Recurrent disease in the remaining gastric pouch may be infiltrative, as shown in Fig. 40, or polypoid (Fig. 41). The pouch inflates quite well with air as a rule, and may be inspected in its entirety. Suspicion of this type of lesion is a prime indication for the use of the previously described Olympus fiberesophagoscope with forward viewing, controllable tip and biopsy forceps, although the longer biopsy fibergastroscopes also perform very satisfactorily. Polypoid cancers of this type may be simulated by large phytobezoars, which occur not uncommonly in the post-resection stomach. The differential in such cases is best made by gastroscopy, and has resulted in successful conservative treatment in several patients in our experience.

Metastatic Carcinoma. Metastatic cancer of the stomach may occur as a result of direct extension from an adjacent organ or tumor mass, or hematologically from a distant primary. Fig. 42 represents penetration of the greater curvature of the antrum from a primary hepatoma, as described in the following case report:

Case Report. A 65-year-old white male was first seen March 1, 1968 with a tumor mass in the epigastrium. This was established by liver biopsy to be hepatoma, and the patient was placed on 5-Fluorouracil therapy. Prior to being placed on therapy, however, he was gastroscoped and a peculiar looking ulcer was noted in the distal antrum which appeared to have something projecting from it (Fig. 42). Six weeks later the polypoid component appeared much more evident at gastroscopy and it was determined that this was a tumor involving the anterior wall of the antrum, which regressed considerably in size on chemotherapy. Metastases were noted to both lungs during the course of the disease and the patient expired three months after the initial diagnosis. Postmortem examination showed carcinoma of the liver, hepatoma with direct invasion of the hepatic vein, liver capsule, diaphragm, gallbladder and stomach and metastases to the lungs.

Malignant melanoma is one of the more frequent invaders of the gastrointestinal tract, especially the stomach. These lesions are usually described radiographically as having a "typical" appearance of umbilicated elevations of the mucosa, which undoubtedly do occur. However, we have not found that melanoma produces metastases which are more "typical" than any others, and the majority have not shown this configuration. The following case report, with findings as illustrated in Figs. 43 and 44, demonstrates this point.

Case Report. A 34-year-old white male was first seen on June 3, 1968 with nodes in the left groin of three months' duration and nausea, particularly when his stomach was empty. There had been weight loss and a biopsy of a left inguinal node had revealed malignant melanoma. The patient showed many subcutaneous nodules, a grayish color to the skin and hepatosplenomegaly. Roentgenograms of stomach and small bowel revealed only a duodenal nodule of undetermined origin. Gastroscopy showed multiple small black metastatic lesions of the stomach (Figs. 43 and 44). He was placed on chemotherapy but repeat gastroscopy failed to show any changes in the gastric lesions. He expired four months later.

Comment: This patient's gastric metastases would have remained undetected except for gastroscopy. Multiple nodular melanotic spread to the stomach is not unusual in this type of malignancy, and often presents no "typical" picture either by roentgenography or gastroscopy. As in most cases treated by chemotherapy, endoscopic examination after a suitable interval represented the only accurate means of appraisal of the results.

Gastric Biopsy. Improved instruments and color photography have added a great deal to endoscopy in gastric cancer, but directed biopsy promises to be the major advance in this field. The technique is relatively easily acquired by the expert endoscopist, and while there are a few pertinent points that must be experienced to be completely appreciated, the ability to biopsy places in the hands of the gastroscopist the ultimate proof—histologic confirmation of neoplasia without the necessity of surgical exploration.

Our modest experience with biopsy in 32 patients with proven cancer, while hardly worthy of comparison with the extensive work done by the Japanese, confirms their optimistic reports. Positive specimens were obtained in 28 of the 32 patients, for an accuracy of 87 per cent. All but four of these positive specimens were obtained at the initial examination, allowing a 24-hour potential in the identification of gastric cancer, in patients who often had waited weeks or months for clarification of symptoms and/or abnormal roentgenological findings. This experience during the past 15 months has been most impressive, and is one of the main points we hope to publicize in this monograph. When better biopsy forceps are available, and we have had the opportunity to use guided-stream washing for gastric cytology in suspicious but biopsy-negative stomachs, it may well be that overall results will be similar to those reported by KASUGAI (1969), and others in Japan (see Chapter 2).

In summary, it should be realized that gastroscopy, once considered supplementary to roentgenoscopic examination in gastric cancer, should now be rated as complementary and equal in the role of diagnosis. Statements such as "in patients suspected of antral malignancy on the basis of x-ray examination, the endoscopic examination is not sufficiently dependable to rule it out", and "Roentgen-ray study is necessary to the diagnosis of almost every case and gastroscopy is not essential if the x-ray findings are conclusive" no longer hold. Cancer may be ruled out or in by gastroscopy and biopsy of the antrum, and "conclusive" x-ray findings have proven erroneous, even when the procedure was performed by highly-qualified radiologists. When not carried out by experienced personnel, as is frequently the case outside of academic institutions which provide most of the statistical studies, roentgenograms may be quite inaccurate and misleading in producing the phantom tumor as well as in missing the bonafide lesion.

Both x-ray and gastroscopic examinations should be performed in all patients suspected of having gastric cancer. The importance of making the correct diagnosis is too great, and the chance of error when only one of these procedures is employed too high, for either to be omitted. Added to these considerations is the present ability to confirm the diagnosis histologically by endoscopy in 80 to 90 per cent of gastric cancer. The routine complementary use of these two procedures, when adopted more generally, will promote earlier and more accurate diagnosis in this field.

Lymphoma

Leiomyosarcoma and malignant lymphoma represent a very small proportion of malignant gastric tumors, approximately 3—4 per cent. They have a relatively more optimistic prognosis when properly treated, and although most of the primary tumors are resected, radiation and chemotherapy may be successfully employed in some when surgical resection is contraindicated. When the lymphoma is generalized, and gastric involvement incidental, radiation or chemotherapy may be the treatment of choice.

The differentiation of this type of neoplasia from carcinoma may therefore be of some importance in the individual patient. Despite these considerations, and even though the accurate diagnosis of leiomyosarcoma and lymphoma is generally impossible by roentgenoscopy, gastroscopy has been seldom employed. The studies of FRAZER (1959), MARSHALL and MEISSNER (1950), WELBORN et al. (1965), WOLFERTH et al. (1959), SNODDY (1952), FAVIS and SALTZSTEIN (1964), OCHSNER and OCHSNER (1955), and JENSEN (1967) do not mention gastroscopy, nor do the comprehensive reviews of DIXON and SHONYO (1949) or FERRIS (1964). In several small groups of five to ten patients each with lymphoma, endoscopy was carried out in single individuals without a correct diagnosis (CULVER et al., 1955; MALEY, 1959; GARVIE, 1965; SWAIN, 1961; TAYLOR, 1939; McNEER and BERG, 1959). In other larger studies by THORBJARNARSON et al. (1956, 1959), JOSEPH and LATTES (1966), JACOBS (1963), TESLER (1959), RUFFIN (1950), and FRIEDMAN (1959), up to 20 per cent of all patients were gastroscoped, with a few positive diagnoses. The general results, however, seemed slightly poorer than roentgenoscopy in differentiating carcinoma from lymphoma.

Because of a rather larger than average number of gastric lymphomas and sarcomas available on the services of our institution, with excellent intraservice cooperation in referral for consultation, a 10 year prospective study was carried out to determine whether gastroscopy and color photography would add appreciably to the accuracy of gross diagnosis of this type of neoplasia. At the end of this period, information had been obtained on 29 patients, of whom 17 had primary gastric lesions (six with leiomyosarcoma, six with lymphosarcoma, and five with reticulum cell sarcoma), and 12 with systemic lymphoma with stomach involvement (eight lymphosarcoma, two reticulum cell sarcoma, and two Hodgkin's disease). Expert radiological examination, gastroscopy and gastroscopic color photographs were obtained in all patients. In addition, eight patients with leiomyoma were studied in the same manner, because of the obvious similarity of the gastroscopic findings in this tumor and leiomyosarcoma (NELSON, 1968).

The results in general with either gastroscopy or roentgenoscopy were not promising. Gastroscopy performed better in leiomyoma and leiomyosarcoma. Leiomyoma was firmly diagnosed in three cases by gastroscopy, in none by roentgenoscopy. Leiomyosarcoma was undiagnosed by either method, although gastroscopically lymphoma was indicated in two cases, carcinoma in two, and leiomyoma in one. Radiographically, carcinoma was described in two of these six patients, and the tumor was not seen in the remaining four. In the primary lymphoma group, roentgenoscopy performed more satisfactorily than gastroscopy, with a firm diagnosis of lymphoma in five, carcinoma in five, and a single patient in whom the tumor was missed. Only one patient was diagnosed as sarcoma by gastroscopy, carcinoma was noted in five, undiagnosed tumor in two, inflammatory changes in two, and a deformed antrum in one. In the group of systemic lymphoma with stomach involvement gastroscopy diagnosed the disease in all but one instance, but this accuracy must be viewed with some reservations in light of the fact that the diagnosis of generalized disease was known to the endoscopist at the time of examination. However, with this prior information, the lesions were visualized and most of them photographed. Roentgenoscopy did not fare so well, possibly because of poorer information. Lymphoma was diagnosed in seven patients, carcinoma in two, benign ulcers in one, and no lesions were visualized in the remaining two patients.

With this somewhat spotty record, gastroscopic photographs were viewed retrospectively with a view to determining what characteristics, if any, would allow the differentiation between carcinoma and lymphoma. It was found that most lymphomas were diffuse and infiltrating, with frequent ulcerations, and when these were the gross characteristics, the differential was impossible. Only two categories, leiomyosarcoma and reticulum cell sarcoma, presented any real possibilities of "typical" gross lesions capable of identifying the individual tumors, and these occurred in only a certain number of each.

Leiomyosarcomas were found to present as submucosal, smooth tumor masses, either uni- or multi-lobed, with normal-appearing surrounding mucosa, and frequently one or more ulcerations at the apex. It was impossible to determine the extragastric component, which was frequently considerable. Since the tumor was submucosal, gastroscopy appeared to visualize the tumor better than roentgenoscopy.

Reticulum cell sarcoma, although diffusely infiltrating, had a tendency in some patients to produce a peculiar volcano-like projection with ulcerated top—a "crater ulcer"—which was found in no other type of lymphoma. This observation still holds true. Of 15 reticulum cell sarcomas, 13 of which were studied on our service and two seen in consultation, seven exhibited this characteristic finding. The "crater ulcer" is well shown in Fig. 45 (early and late stage of development), and the course of the disease illustrated by the case report of this patient.

Case Report. This 63-year-old white female was first seen August 6, 1968 complaining of epigastric pain accompanied by nausea, vomiting and hematemesis for a period of two months, as well as severe melena. A roentgenogram accompanying her taken one month previously showed a constant irregular contour defect in the antrum of the stomach with a superficial ulceration. At gastroscopy the antrum seemed to be grossly involved with submucosal tumor. There was some necrosis on the posterior wall and on the anterior wall of the stomach were two raised discrete ulcer craters (Fig. 45). Their general appearance was that of gastric lymphoma, probably reticulum cell sarcoma. Two biopsies were taken which showed unclassified malignant neoplasm, probably reticulum cell sarcoma (Figs. 45a and 45b). The patient was feeble-minded and did not desire surgery for her disease. She was therefore placed on cytoxan and repeat examination showed marked extension of necrosis, probably as result of this drug. There were huge ulcerations of the body of the stomach with evidence of massive bleeding. She continued to bleed, went into shock and expired September 23, 1968. Autopsy showed acute peritonitis secondary to perforated reticulum cell sarcoma which involved stomach, left kidney and gastric lymph nodes. The cause of death was attributed to clostridial septicemia.

The remainder of these lesions were massively infiltrating, sometimes ulcerated, and could not be distinguished from other lymphomas or carcinoma. The massively infiltrating type is represented by Fig. 46, a patient who was treated with radiation with excellent results, and the massively ulcerating feature is shown in another patient as noted in Fig. 47.

Diffuse infiltration may also be a feature of lymphocytic lymphoma, as seen in the spectacular example in Fig. 48. The case report of this patient is given below.

Case Report. This 42-year-old white female was first seen June 23, 1966 complaining of easy fatigability and a maculopapular rash over the entire body with pruritus for two months. There had been a 12 pound weight loss and a mass found in the left upper quadrant. Chest x-ray showed hilar adenopathy. Biopsies taken from cervical nodes on the left showed lymphocytic lymphoma, poorly differentiated, either lymphoma or reticulum cell sarcoma. X-rays showed extreme distortion of the stomach with large lobular masses arising from various mucosal areas of the stomach. Gastroscopy confirmed this picture. One of the massive submucosal infiltrates was ulcerated and it was felt that the picture was more typical of lymphoma than carcinoma. The patient received irradiation to the upper abdomen as well as chemotherapy. She did quite well over a period of two years but then expired of her disease.

Another case, with marked hemorrhagic-type infiltrates and a peculiar flat ulceration, is seen in Fig. 49.

Two additional illustrations are included because of their rarity, although there is nothing about the gross characteristics of these two tumors which would render them diagnosable at gastroscopy. The peculiar nodular elevation, with multi-nodular infiltrates involving a large part of the stomach distally (Fig. 50), was photographed in a patient with multiple myeloma, later found at autopsy to have myelomatous infiltrates of the stomach. Such involvement is extremely rare in systemic multiple myeloma. Fig. 51 demonstrates the large, meaty appearance assumed by some rapidly growing sarcomas in the stomach (in this case a rare neurogenic sarcoma).

The limited clues as to differentiation of lymphoma from carcinoma appeared to invalidate any claim that gastroscopy would help particularly in preoperative diagnosis of these lesions. Insofar as gross features are concerned, this is still true. However, another diagnostic modality has recently become available to us which has radically altered the picture. This is directed gastric biopsy.

Gastric Biopsy. Cytology following gastric lavage, fairly successful in our hands in adenocarcinoma of the stomach, has appeared to be almost useless in lymphoma. There was some question, also, as to whether the small specimen obtained with presently available instruments would be adequate for definite pathological interpretation. Despite these misgivings, all available lymphomas of the stomach have been biopsied under direct vision during the past 18 months.

The preliminary results have been uniformly good. Six patients biopsied prior to surgical resection or radiation were all positive on the first attempt, and while there was some hedging by the pathologists, could be identified as lymphoma. A typical example is given in the case report already presented, whose gastroscopic photograph is shown in Fig. 45, and biopsy specimens in Figs. 45a and 45b. In addition, four patients have been biopsied following treatment for gastric lymphoma, two of whom were seen postoperatively, and two after receiving radiation. Gross inspection of the stomach or remaining stomach pouch combined with multiple negative biopsies and careful follow-up have confirmed the efficacy of treatment in all four cases. We now feel that in selected patients in whom there is a contraindication to surgery, radiation may be given without open biopsy on the basis of gastroscopic examination and directed biopsy. An illustrative case report follows (gastroscopic photograph shown in Fig. 46).

Case Report. A 52-year-old white female was seen on June 24, 1968 with symptoms of weakness, fever and some epigastric distress. Roentgenograms had shown probable tumor of the stomach. It was felt that the findings were those of lymphoma but there was no evidence of extragastric mass. At gastroscopy, the entire stomach surface appeared to be infiltrated submucosally with large folds and polypoid masses, one of which was ulcerated and bleeding. The majority of the involvement seemed to be in the fundus along the greater curvature and posterior wall. On June 27, 1968, esophagoscopy was done and several biopsies of the stomach obtained through the esophagoscope. These were read as showing histiocytic reticulum cell sarcoma. The patient was placed on x-ray therapy to the stomach and abdominal nodes. A total of 4,000 rads were given to the left upper quadrant and 3,000 rads to the entire upper abdomen. Treatment was completed September 7, 1968, following which the patient did well. Follow-up x-ray studies showed almost complete disappearance of the large folds in the upper stomach. There was a narrowing at the midportion but no definite evidence of tumor could be seen. On the last study two small ulcerations were noted by x-ray. Gastroscopic follow-up was carried out on two occasions five months apart following therapy. There appeared to be some large folds but no definite tumor could be made out and most of the stomach showed no evidence of tumor. Biopsies taken on both of these occasions were read as essentially normal mucosa. The patient has gained weight and felt quite well on continued follow-up.

This small number of cases is only a modest beginning, and because of their scarcity it will be some years before the exact status of gastroscopy and guided biopsy in lymphoma can be determined. However, it appears that biopsy is at least as accurate in this type of neoplasia as in carcinoma, and the ability to make a presurgical histological diagnosis may be even more valuable in lymphoma. The recommendation can be made that as in carcinoma, all cases with roentgen or other evidence of primary disease should have gastroscopy. In patients with generalized lymphoma, gastroscopy should be employed in all those with upper gastrointestinal symptoms regardless of whether or not there is radiological evidence of disease, since the early stage of stomach involvement may not be detected by x-ray examination.

Summary

The development of more flexible and maneuverable instruments coupled with the ability to make color photographs of gastric lesions and take guided biopsies under gastroscopic observation, have altered the clinical management of patients with lesions suspected of being possible cancer. The great majority of gastric ulcers may be accurately diagnosed as benign or malignant prior to surgery on the basis of gross and microscopic features, and a blanket policy of resection in all cases is unjustified. The natural history of gastritis and gastropathies is slowly being clarified, and their differentiation from carcinoma or lymphoma can be made in most patients.

Gastric polyps are better visualized by gastroscopy, and concurrent cancer can now be diagnosed by biopsy in such patients, although biopsy of the individual small polyp has been disappointing. Carcinoma and lymphoma are best studied through the gastroscope, and both can be biopsied with a high degree of accuracy. In some patients with lymphoma, particularly the generalized type, positive biopsy makes treatment with radiation or chemotherapy possible without the necessity of surgical exploration.

References

ARIGA, K., HONDA, T., TANAKA, S.: The follow-up studies on the endoscopic finding of gastric ulcer. Proceedings of the First Congress of the International Society of Endoscopy. Tokyo (Japan): Hitachi Printing Co. 1967, p. 277.

BALFOUR, D. C., HIGHTOWER, N. C., GAMBILL, E. E., WAUGH, J. M., DOCKERTY, M. B.: Giant hypertrophy of the gastric rugae (Menetrier's disease) associated with severe hypo-proteinemia relieved only by total gastrectomy: report of case. Gastroenterology 16, 773 (1950).

BUTZ, W. C.: Giant hypertrophic gastritis. Gastroenterology 39, 183 (1960).

CAREY, J. B., HAY, L.: Gastric polyps. Gastroenterology 10, 102 (1948).

CHARLES, R. N., MOSS, A. J., KUNZ, W., SEGAL, H. L.: Gastric secretory derangement in Menetrier's disease. Amer. J. dig. Dis. 8, 192 (1963).

CHUSID, E. L., HIRSCH, R. L., COLCHER, H.: Spectrum of hypertrophic gastropathy: giant fugal folds, polyposis, and carcinoma of the stomach—case report and review of the literature. Arch. int. Med. 114, 621 (1964).

CITRIN, Y., STERLING, K., HALSTED, J. A.: The mechanism of hypoproteinemia associated with giant hypertrophy of the gastric mucosa. New Engl. J. Med. 257, 906 (1957).

COHEN, N. N., HUGHES, R. W., MANFREDO, H. E.: Experience with 1,000 fiber gastroscopic examinations of the stomach. Amer. J. dig. Dis. 11, 943 (1966).

CULVER, G. J., BEAN, B. C., BERENS, D. L.: Gastric lymphoma. Radiology 65, 518 (1955).

DiBIANCO, J., NISSENBAUM, G., ATTIA, A., GROSSIER, V. W.: Multiple polyps of the stomach: a cinefiber-gastroscopic study. Bull. Gastroint. Endosc. 11, 10 (1965).

DIXON, C. F., SHONYO, E. S.: Differential diagnosis of sarcoma of the stomach. Surg. Clin. N. Amer. August 1949, p. 1109.

DODD, G. D., NELSON, R. S.: The combined radiologic and gastroscopic evaluation of gastric ulceration. Radiology 77, 177 (1961).

FAVIS, T. D., SALZSTEIN, S. L.: Gastric lymphoid hyperplasia: a lesion confused with lym-phosarcoma. Cancer 17, 207 (1964).

FERRIS, D. A.: Gastric Sarcoma in Cancer of the Stomach. Philadelphia (Pa.): W. B. Saunders Co. 1964, p. 158.

FIEBER, S. S.: Hypertrophic gastritis. Gastroenterology 28, 29 (1955).

FRAZER, J. W., JR.: Malignant lymphomas of the gastrointestinal tract. Surg. Gynec. Obstet. 108, 182 (1959).

FRIEDMAN, A. I.: Primary lymphosarcoma of the stomach. A clinical study of seventy-five cases. Amer. J. Med. 26, 783 (1959).

GAMES, A. D., HAWK, W. A., OWENS, F. J., BROWN, C. H.: Hypertrophic gastropathy and carcinoma of the stomach. Gastroint. Endosc. 12, 29 (1966).

GARRY, M. W.: A patient with multiple gastric polyps observed over a ten year period. Bull. Gastrosc. and Esophagosc. 5, 6 (1959).

GARVIS, W. H. H.: Leiomyosarcoma of the stomach. Brit. J. Surg. 52, 32 (1965).

JACOBS, D. S.: Primary gastric malignant lymphoma and pseudo-lymphoma. Amer. J. clin. Path. 40, 370 (1963).

JENSEN, F. B.: Primary gastric sarcoma. Acta chir. scand. 133, 139 (1967).

JONES, F. A., GUMMER, J. W. P.: Clinical Gastroenterology. Springfield (Ill.): Charles C Thomas 1960, p. 256.

JOSEPH, J. I., LATTES, R.: Gastric lymphosarcoma. Amer. J. clin. Path. 45, 653 (1966).

KASUGAI, T.: Endoscopy in Japan with special reference to detection of gastric cancer. Gastroint. Endosc. 51, 204 (1969).

KENNEY, F. D., DOCKERTY, M. S., WAUGH, J. M.: Giant hypertrophy of the gastric mucosa. Cancer 7, 671 (1954).

KONJEZTNY, G. E.: Der Magenkrebs. Stuttgart: F. Eulse 1938.

MAIMON, S. N., BARTLESS, J. P., HUMPHREYS, E. M., PALMER, W. L.: Giant hypertrophic gastritis. Gastroenterology 8, 397 (1947).

MARSHALL, S. F., MEISSNER, W. A.: Sarcoma of the stomach. Ann. Surg. 131, 824 (1950).

MASLEY, P. M.: Leiomyosarcoma of the stomach. Amer. J. dig. Dis. 4, 792 (1959).

MATZNER, M. J., RAAB, A. P., SPEAR, P. W.: Benign giant gastric rugae complicated by submucosal gastric carcinoma. Gastroenterology 18, 296 (1951).

McNEER, G., BERG, J. W.: The clinical behavior and management of primary malignant lymphoma of the stomach. Surgery 46, 829 (1959).

— PACK, G. T.: Neoplasms of the Stomach. Philadelphia (Pennsylvania): J. P. Lippincott Co. 1967, p. 222.

MENETRIER, P.: Des polyadenomas gastriques et de leurs rapports avec le cancer de l'estomac. Arch. de physiol. norm. et path. s. 41, 236 (1888).

MONAGHAN, J. F., NAST, P. R.: In: Gastroenterology, Vol. 1. Ed.: H. L. BOCKUS. Philadelphia (Pennsylvania): W. B. Saunders Co. 1963, p. 523.

MORAN, J. M., BEAL, J. M.: Giant hypertrophic gastritis. Amer. J. Surg. 98, 584 (1959).

NELSON, R. S.: Gastroscopic experiences in the United States Army, Europe. Amer. J. dig. Dis. 21, 128 (1954).

— Myoepithelial hamartoma of the stomach. Bull. Gastrosc. and Esophagosc. 6, 24 (1959).

— Gastroscopic observation on the persimmon bezoar. Bull. Gastroint. Endosc. 10, 9 (1963).

— Gastroscopic Photography. Chicago (Ill.): Year Book Med. Publ. 1966, p. 58.

— LANZA, F. L.: Endoscopy in the diagnosis of gastric lymphoma and sarcoma. Amer. J. Gastroent. 50, 37 (1968).

— SCOTT, N. M.: Heterotopic pancreatic tissue in the stomach, gastroscopic features. Gastroenterology 34, 452 (1958).

OCHSNER, S., OCHSNER, A.: Sarcoma of the stomach. Ann. Surg. 142, 804 (1955).

OLSEN, A. M.: Gastroscopic Diagnosis in Cancer of the Stomach. Philadelphia (Pa.): W. B. Saunders Co. 1964, p. 40.

PALMER, E. D.: Gastric adenomas: polyps and polyposis. Stomach Disease as Diagnosed by Gastroscopy. Philadelphia (Pa.): Lea and Febiger 1949.

— Gastroscopic experiences with benign gastric tumours. Bull. Gastroint. Endosc. 11, 16 (1965).

PALMER, W. L.: In: A textbook of medicine. Eds.: CECIL and LOEB. Philadelphia (Pa.): W. B. Saunders Co. 1959, p. 808.

PAUL, W. D., LOGAN, W. P.: Polyps of the stomach with reference to gastroscopic findings. Gastroenterology 8, 592 (1947).

ReMINE, W. H., PRIESTLEY, J. T., BERKSON, J.: Cancer of the Stomach. Philadelphia (Pa.): W. B. Saunders Co. 1964, p. 42.

RUFFIN, J.: Primary lymphosarcoma of the stomach with five-year survival after operation; clinical, x-ray and gastroscopic features. Gastroenterology 16, 250 (1950).

SAKITA, T., TAKASU, S., OMORI, K., FUKUTOMI, H.: On the clinical course of the gastric ulcer. Proceedings of the First Congress of the International Society of Endoscopy. Tokyo (Japan): Hitachi Printing Co. 1967, p. 280.

SATO, K., WADA, T.: Serial gastrofiberscopic observations of gastric ulcer. Proceedings of the First Congress of the International Society of Endoscopy. Tokyo (Japan): Hitachi Printing Co. 1967, p. 344.

SCHINDLER, R.: Gastritis. New York: Grune & Stratton 1947.

— DESNEUX, J. J.: Gastroscopic diagnosis in 273 gastric ulcers. Gastroenterology 24, 328 (1953).

SLEISENGER, M. H.: In: Principles of Internal Medicine. Ed.: T. R. HARRISON. New York: McGraw-Hill Book Co. 1962, p. 1611.

SNODDY, W. T.: Primary lymphosarcoma of the stomach. Gastroenterology 20, 537 (1952).

SPELLBERG, M. A., BAKER, L.: Gastritis: its clinical significance. Med. Clin. N. Amer. 37, 41 (1953).

STOUT, A. P.: Pathology of carcinoma of the stomach. Arch. Surg. **46**, 807 (1943).
— Tumors of the Stomach. Atlas of Tumor Pathology, Section VI. Fasc. 21. Washington: Armed Forces of Pathology 1953.
— Foreword. In: Neoplasms of the Stomach. Eds.: G. McNEER and G. T. PACK. Philadelphia (Pa.): J. B. Lippincott Co. 1967.
SWAIN, J.: Sarcoma of the stomach of lymphoid origin. Med. J. Aust. **11**, 479 (1961).
TAYLOR. E. S.: Primary lymphosarcoma of the stomach. Ann. Surg. **110**, 200 (1939).
TESLER, J.: Primary lymphosarcoma of the stomach. Amer. J. Gastroent. **32**, 557 (1959).
TEXTER, E. C., LEGERTON, C. W., REEVES, R. J., SMITH, A. G., RUFFIN, J. M.: Coexistent carcinoma of the stomach and hypertrophic gastritis. Gastroenterology **24**, 579 (1953).
THORBJARNARSON, B., BEAL, J. M., PEARCE, J. M.: Primary malignant lymphoid tumors of the stomach. Cancer **9**, 712 (1956).
— PEARCE, J. M., BEAL, J. M.: Sarcoma of the stomach. Amer. J. Surg. **97**, 36 (1959).
UTSUMI, Y., MIWA, T., FUJINO, M., YOSHITOSHI, Y.: Prognosis of gastric ulcer—its healing and recurrence. Proceedings of the First Congress of the International Society of Endoscopy. Tokyo (Japan): Hitachi Printing Co. 1967, p. 138.
V. A. Gastric Ulcer Study Group. The Veterans Administration Cooperative Study on Gastric Ulcer: Healing, Recurrence. Cancer Gastroenterology (abstract) **56**, 1208 (1969).
WELBORN, J. K., PONKA, J. L., REBUCK, J. W.: Lymphoma of the stomach. Arch. Surg. **90**, 480 (1965).
WOLFERTH, C. C., JR., BRADY, L. W., ENTERLINE, H. T., BLAKEMORE, W. S.: Primary lymphosarcoma of the stomach. Surg. Gynec. Obstet. **109**, 755 (1959).
YARNIS, H., MARSHAK, R. H., FRIEDMAN, A. I.: Gastric polyps. J. Amer. med. Ass. **148**, 1088 (1952).

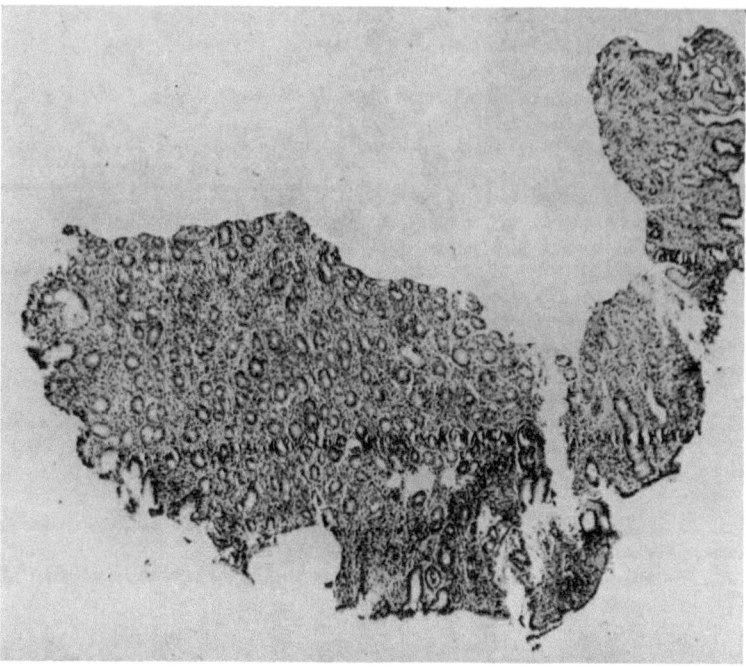

Fig. 9 a. Low-power view of gastric biopsy with marked gastritis, taken from edge of benign ulcer (Fig. 9)

Fig. 7. This small, sharply punched-out ulceration of the anterior wall of the antrum illustrates the characteristics of the typical benign ulcer. There is very little inflammatory reaction, indicative of a healing phase

Fig. 8. The angulus is the frequent seat of ulceration. The lesion shown is not round, but the edges are sharp. Although the mucosa exhibits inflammatory change, there is no evidence of nodularity or tumor. This ulcer was benign on biopsy, but failed to heal and subtotal resection confirmed the biopsy report

Fig. 9. This benign-appearing ulcer, not visualized on roentgenoscopy, was photographed at gastroscopy in a patient with multiple myeloma, and treated with cytosine arabinoside. Another ulcer, which had been diagnosed radiologically, was seen at the same examination (Fig. 12). A biopsy taken from the ulcer edge showed gastritic changes, but no cancer (Fig. 9 a).

Fig. 10. A typical large, sharply punched-out ulceration of the lesser curvature just proximal to the angulus, exhibiting marked inflammatory changes at the margins, severe edema, and converging folds on the posterior wall. Peristaltic waves may be seen traversing the floor of the antrum inferiorly, and puckered folds visible indicate closing of the pylorus (not seen)

Fig. 11. A large (3—4 cm) flat ulceration of the lesser curvature has sharply demarcated edges, and inflammation is indicated by marked edema of the surrounding mucosa. The floor of the crater is covered by bile-stained mucus. Large ulcers of this type, while obviously benign, heal poorly

Fig. 12. The crater of this large, well-demarcated ulcer of the lesser curvature is filled with a clot, which protrudes slightly. The larger of two ulcers seen at gastroscopy (the other shown in Fig. 9), it failed to heal on medical therapy. The poor general condition of the patient precluded surgical intervention, the ulcer perforated, and death due to peritonitis followed

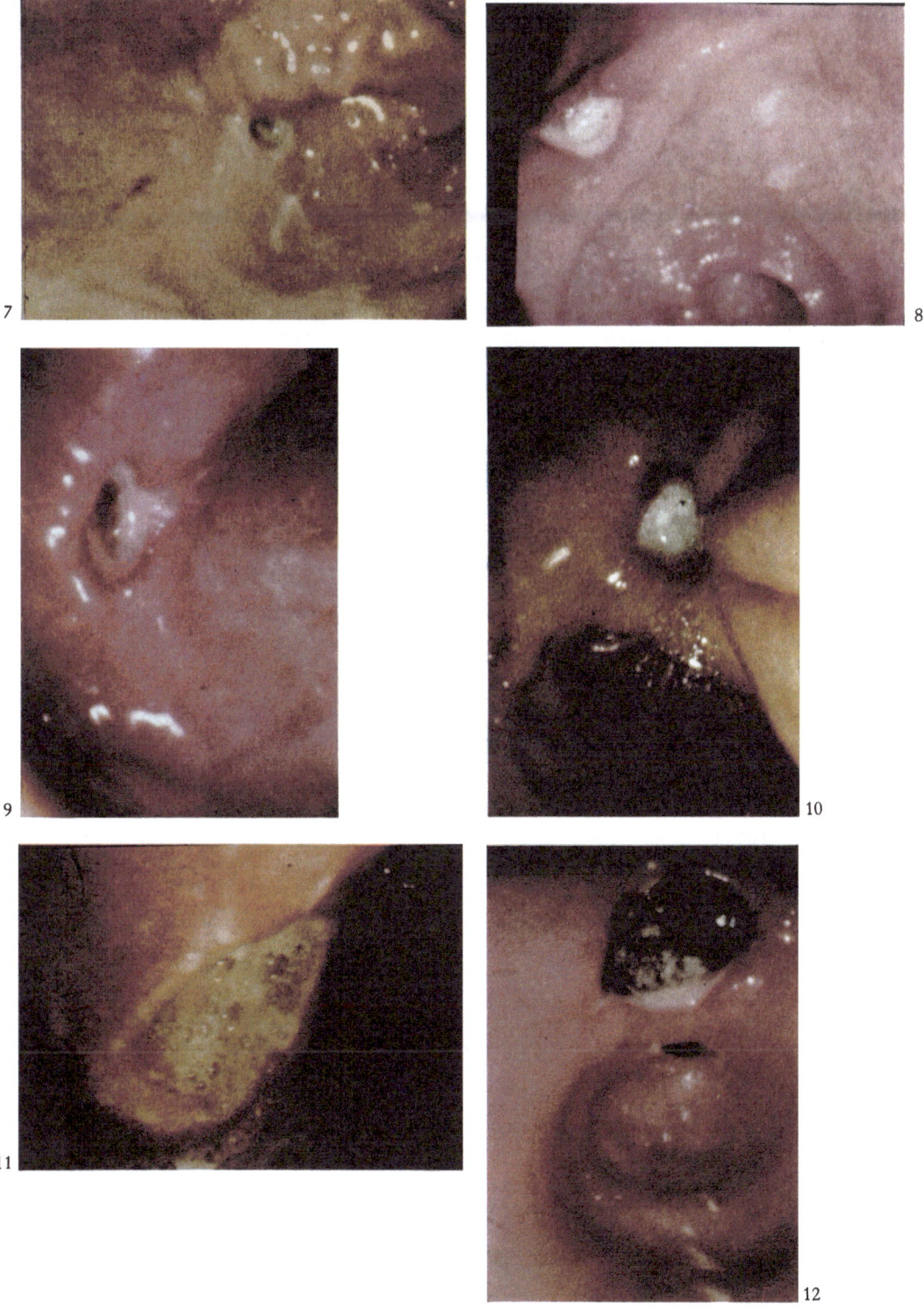

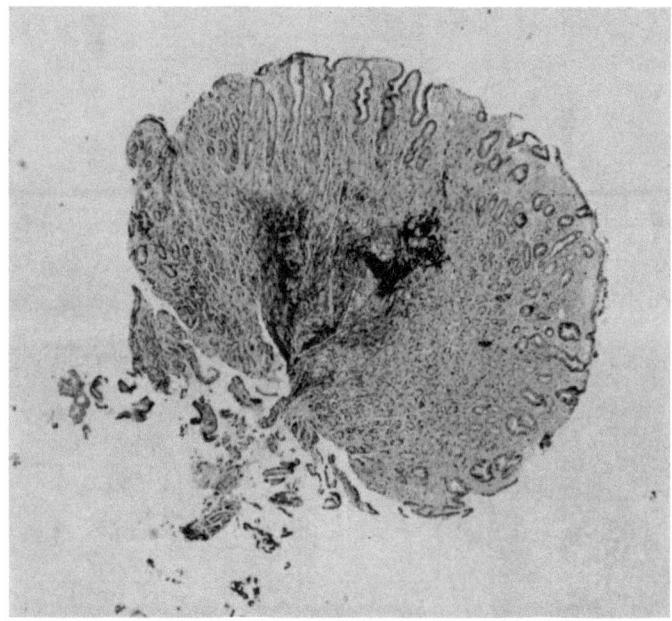

Fig. 18 a. Low-power view of the gastric biopsy from the ulcer shown in Fig. 18. There is
massive inflammatory infiltration and surface gastritis

Fig. 13. This large benign ulcer of the lesser curvature was seen at gastroscopy in a patient
with inoperable cancer of the rectum who had been receiving weekly 5-Fluorouracil
therapy, and developed melena. Evidence of recent bleeding may be seen in the crater of
the ulcer. No healing occurred during a four months' observation period, and the ulcer
itself exhibited little or no change. The generally poor condition of the patient prevented
surgical intervention

Fig. 14. Marked inflammatory changes are noted in the gastric mucosa of the whole
stomach, with an ulceration shown only as a depressed area covered by clot. The patient
responded rapidly to medical therapy as noted by the appearance of the ulcer in Fig. 15

Fig. 15. The same stomach as that shown in Fig. 14. Gastritic changes have subsided after
three weeks' therapy, revealing a benign, healing ulceration of the lesser curvature.
Recovery was eventually complete

Fig. 16. This large, flat-appearing ulceration, surrounded by nodular infiltrates, is typical
of the usual malignant ulceration developing in carcinoma. There is bleeding from the
nodular area to the right of the ulcer, a frequent characteristic of cancer

Fig. 17. This carcinomatous ulcer exhibits the same general appearance as that of the
ulcer in Fig. 16. There is obvious ulceration of a large intragastric mass, the appearance of
which is typical of carcinoma. Gastroscopically, such ulcers are seldom misinterpreted

Fig. 18. The rather shallow type of ulceration seen at the apex of the convering folds
on the posterior wall of the stomach is unusual because of the tremendous inflammatory
reaction surrounding it. The roentgenograms in this patient were non-diagnostic. The
gastroscopic diagnosis of benign gastric ulcer was supported by biopsy (Fig. 18 a), and
eventual gastric resection which confirmed the diagnosis. Ulcers of this type are often
erroneously designated as malignant by both roentgenoscopy and gastroscopy because
of the tremendous inflammatory reaction surrounding them, the cause of which is obscure

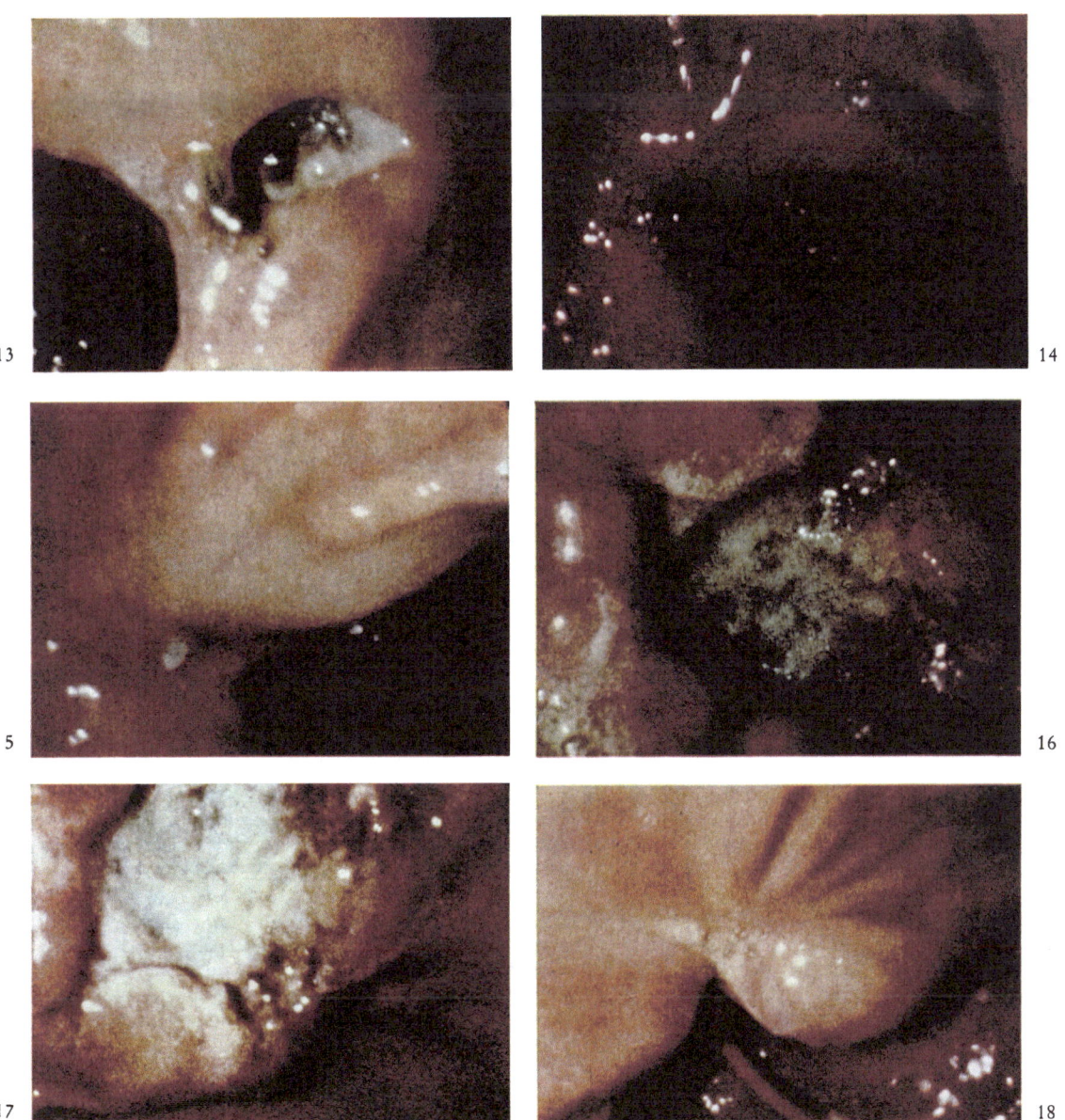

Fig. 19. An 83-year-old white woman had complained of intermittent nausea, vomiting and epigastric pain for several years. Gastroscopy revealed a large, irregular ulceration with marked deformity of the entrance to the antrum and massive infiltration. Biopsies showed only ulceration and inflammation. Surgery was refused. Over a period of 18 months, she has responded symptomatically to medical treatment, but the gastroscopic appearance of the ulcer is unchanged

Fig. 20. A raised, ulcerated area was noted on the greater curvature of the stomach in a 43-year-old man with generalized bone pain, shown on roentgenograms to be due to metastatic cancer. No biopsy was taken due to unavailability of equipment at the time, but opinion was divided as to the nature of this ulcer, which has quite regular edges and no definite nodularity of the mucosa. He deteriorated rapidly, and autopsy revealed the ulcerated area to be cancer of the stomach metastatic to bone

Fig. 21. The gastroscopist's reaction to this ulcer, thought to be benign by roentgenoscopy, was equivocal, although study of the gastroscopic photograph gives definite clues as to its nature. The converging folds are fixed, and appear to be infiltrated. They do not progress up to the crater, but are interrupted in several places, and the crater itself has an irregular margin. Surgical resection carried out because of recurrent bleeding revealed a small ulcerating carcinoma

Fig. 22. The rather shallow, acute ulceration found in this patient's antrum is obviously part of a severe gastritis denoted by reddening, edema, and some fixation of the area surrounding the ulcer (peristaltic waves can be seen progressing through the posterior wall, but not the ulcer area). This type of benign disease has a tendency to become chronic, as shown in Fig. 23

Fig. 23. Antral gastritis has progressed in this instance to marked inflammatory infiltration, deformity of the pylorus, and multiple ulcerations. Many biopsies showed only ulceration and gastritis. Radiographically, this type of antral disease often appears to be carcinoma

Fig. 24. The end results of chronic inflammation, ulceration and scarring of the antrum are evident in this 67-year-old man, who still has a residual ulcer of the angulus super-imposed on a chronic inflammatory background. Nausea, vomiting, and partial obstruction are common; however, the gross picture differs considerably from antral cancer, and we have not observed carcinomatous degeneration on this background (which is not to say it may not occur)

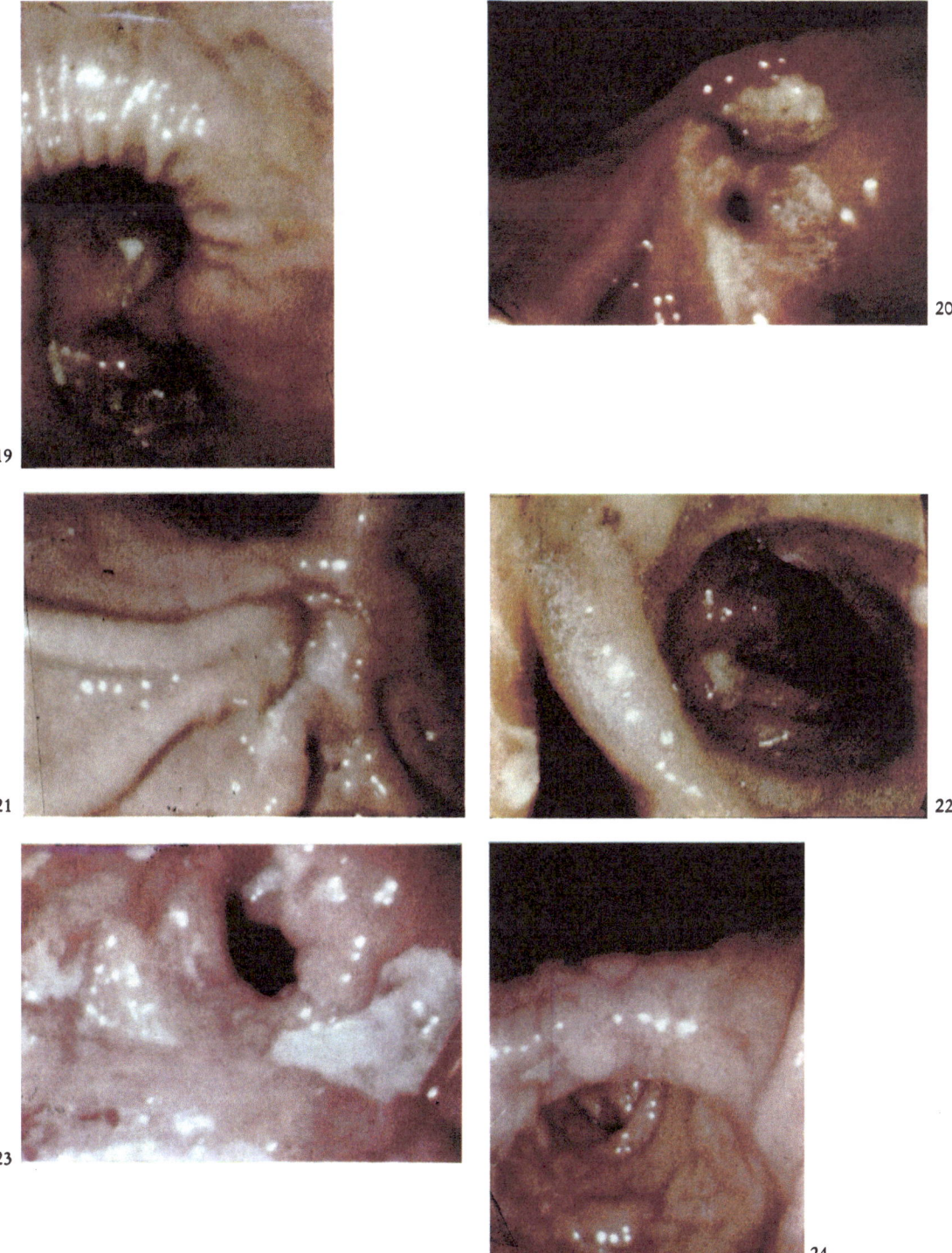

Fig. 25. Multiple hemorrhaging areas ("hemorrhagic gastritis") are clearly visible on the greater curvature of the contracting antrum in a patient with massive upper gastrointestinal hemorrhage. Such changes are found in a significant number of individuals with hemorrhage, and are visible only by gastroscopy. The background mucosa in this patient is pale, evidencing anemia

Fig. 26. The large, irregular, somewhat stiff folds of giant mucosal hypertrophy (Menetrier's disease) are well demonstrated on the greater curvature of this patient's stomach. The disease was first suspected because of protein-losing enteropathy. These changes may be impossible to differentiate from infiltrating carcinoma or lymphoma. There is heavy mucus secretion overlying the surface, also characteristic

Fig. 27. The thickened folds of giant mucosal hypertrophy (proven on open biopsy) are more discrete in this patient, who has been followed gastroscopically over a period of four years. Initially limited to the antral region, the changes have gradually spread to the greater curvature (shown here). Except for hypochromic anemia, there have been few symptoms, and no evidence of complicating carcinoma. Serum proteins have remained normal

Fig. 28. Multiple polyps are visible on a pale background in this stomach. There is bleeding evident high up on the lesser curvature, where there appeared to be some infiltration as well as polyposis, and biopsies were taken. These showed adenocarcinoma (Fig. 28 a and 28 b)

Fig. 29. A large nodular polyp found on the greater curvature side of the fundus (not shown on roentoenograms) in the same stomach as that shown in Fig. 28. There are atrophic changes in the background. Carcinoma, as in this patient, appears to occur more frequently in association with multiple polyposis of the stomach than when the lesion is single

Fig. 30. A single, large, somewhat irregular polyp with a broad base is seen protruding from the greater curvature near the antrum (part of angulus seen in background). Diagnosed as benign by both roentgenoscopy and gastroscopy, this was confirmed on resection

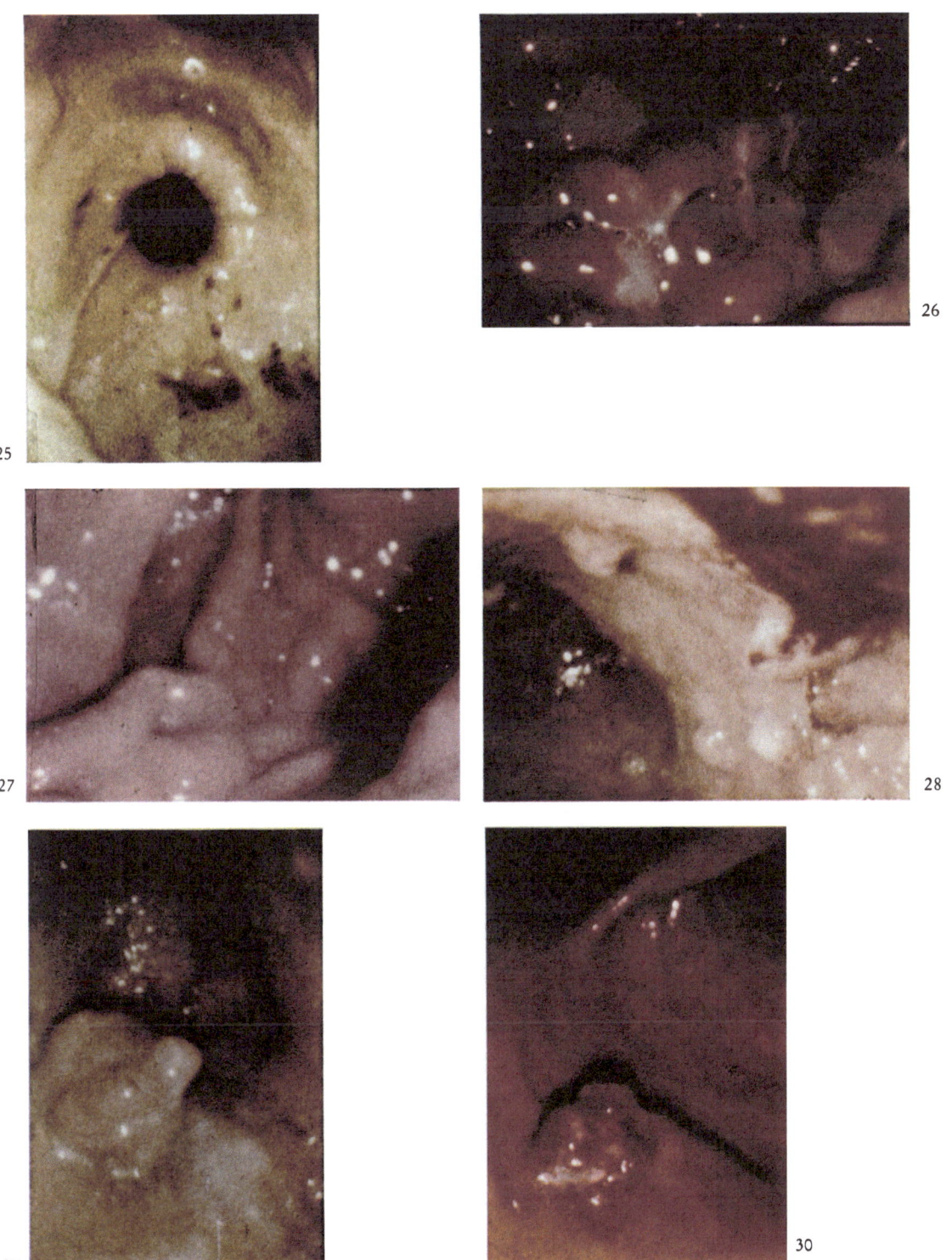

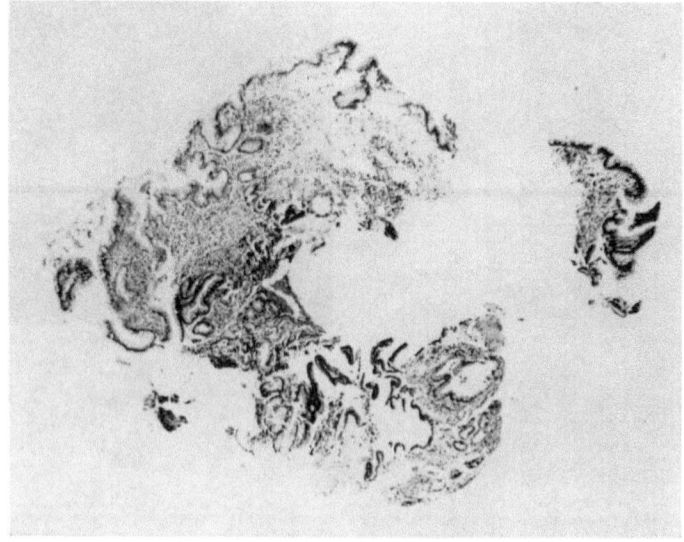

Fig. 28 a. Low-power view of gastroscopic biopsy in patient with multiple polyposis. Carcinomatous change evident

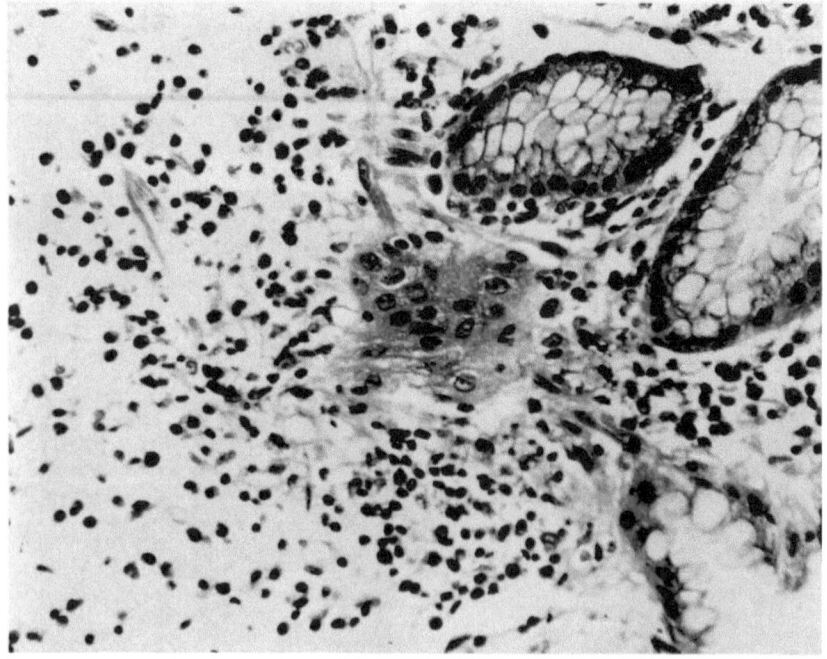

Fig. 28 b. High-power view demonstrates nest of cancer cells in mucosa in same patient as Fig. 28 a

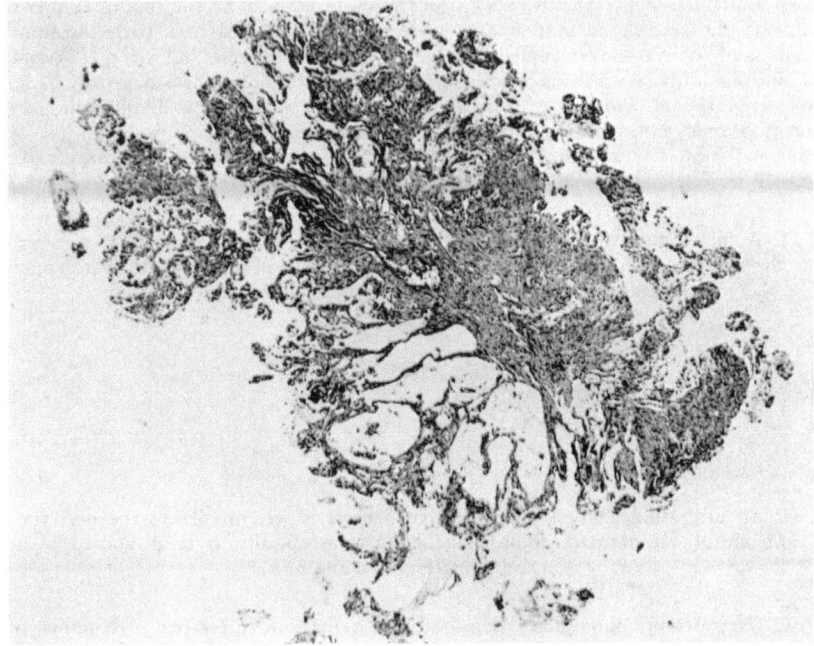

Fig. 33 a. Low-power view shows marked distortion of the mucosal pattern by carcinoma

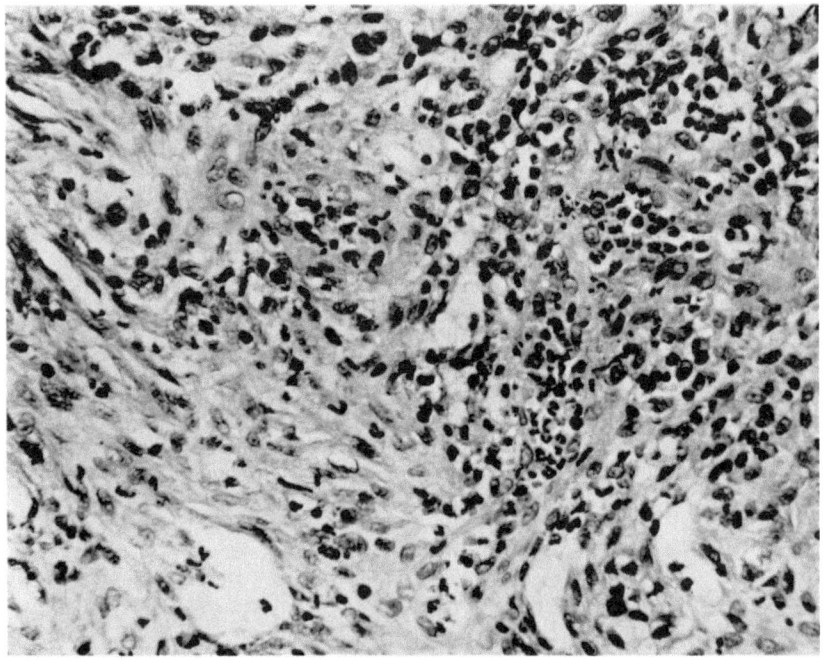

Fig. 33 b. High-power view shows details of invasive carcinoma cells

Fig. 31. A nodular infiltrate can be seen on the posterior wall of the fundus medial to the cardia, on the retroflexed gastroscopic view, in a 49-year-old man with squamous cell carcinoma of the retromolar angle. He had had epigastric distress, and roentgenograms were read unequivocally as showing cancer, which seemed to be confirmed grossly at gastroscopy, even though biopsies of this area showed no malignancy. Exploration revealed marked chronic inflammation involving the liver and posterior wall of the gastric fundus and local nodes. Histologically these resembled sarcoidosis. The stomach was not resected, and seven months later his epigastric distress had disappeared

Fig. 32. A huge, fungating polypoid mass, partly covered with mucus, is seen growing from the anterior wall and lesser curvature of the body of the stomach. The appearance is typical of adenocarcinoma, proved at surgical exploration

Fig. 33. An ulcerating, malignant infiltrative process is seen involving the posterior wall and antrum of the stomach. Biopsies taken gastroscopically were diagnosed as adenocarcinoma (Fig. 33 a and 33 b)

Fig. 34. Gastroscopic photograph demonstrates a massive, ulcerating carcinoma of the lesser curvature of the body and antrum, confirmed at surgical exploration

Fig. 35. A photograph taken in the stomach of a 60-year-old white woman who had had epigastric pain for over three years shows a flat ulcer crater on the apex of what appears to be tumor infiltrate to the left; just below may be seen the greater curvature of the deformed antrum; to the right of this is a massive submucosal tumor with a huge excavating ulceration. Gastroscopic biopsy showed carcinoma. She had surgical removal of both ovaries two years previously for adenocarcinoma, the source of which had not been determined. A palliative resection was performed

Fig. 36. Large folds, apparently the result of submucosal infiltration, are seen in the stomach of a 45-year-old man with a history of gastrointestinal hemorrhage and abdominal pain. The stomach could be only minimally inflated, as shown, and no recognizable ulcer or tumor was unequivocally demonstrated. Gastroscopic biopsies revealed carcinoma
(Fig. 36 a and 36 b)

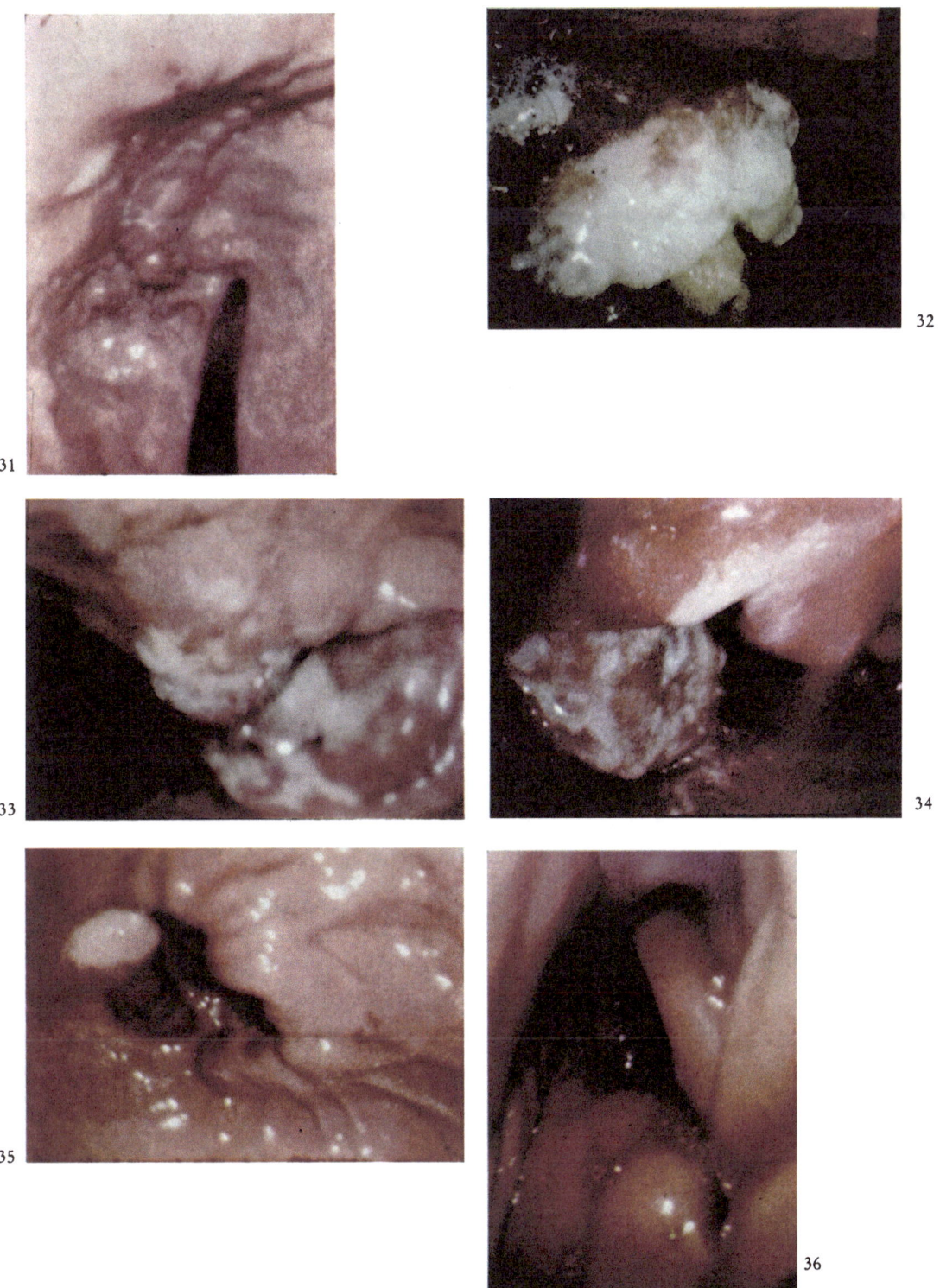

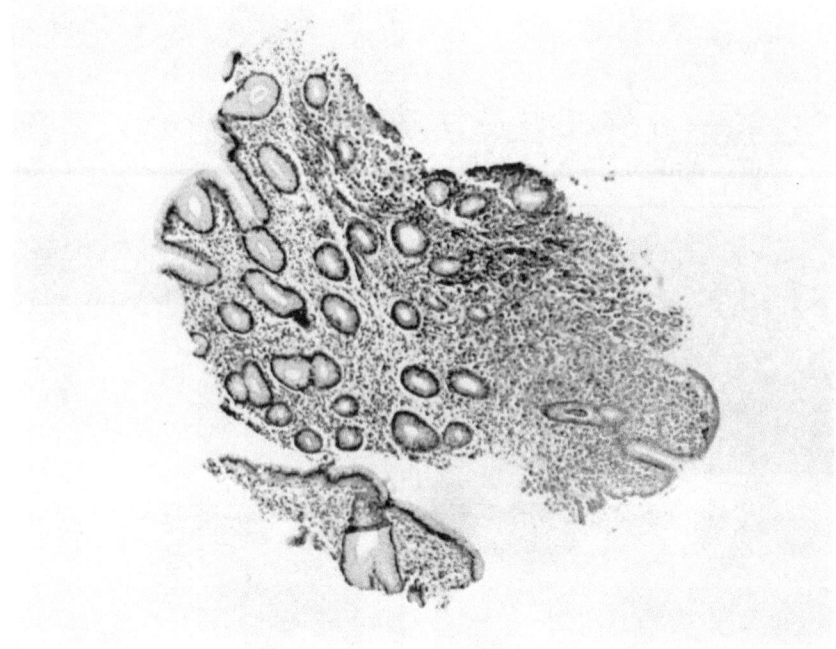

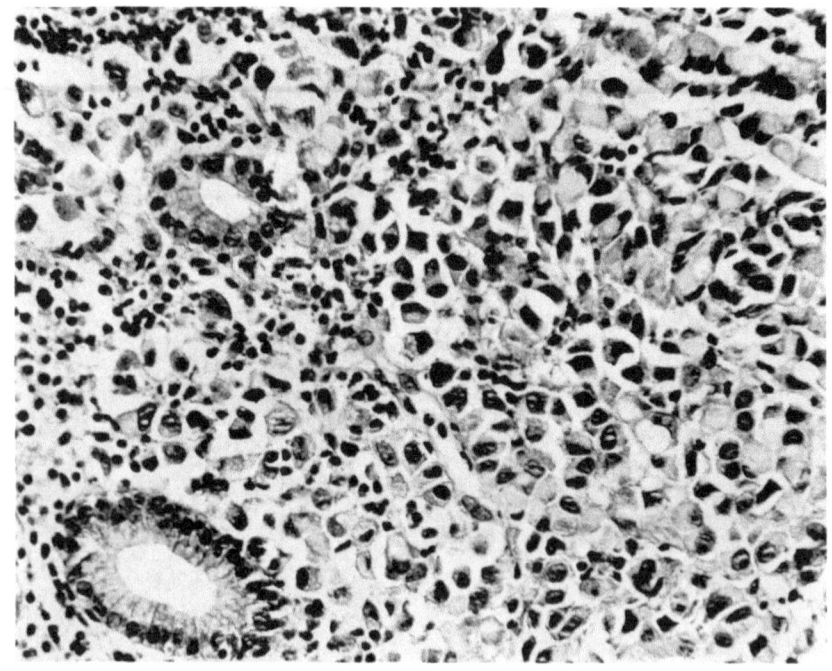

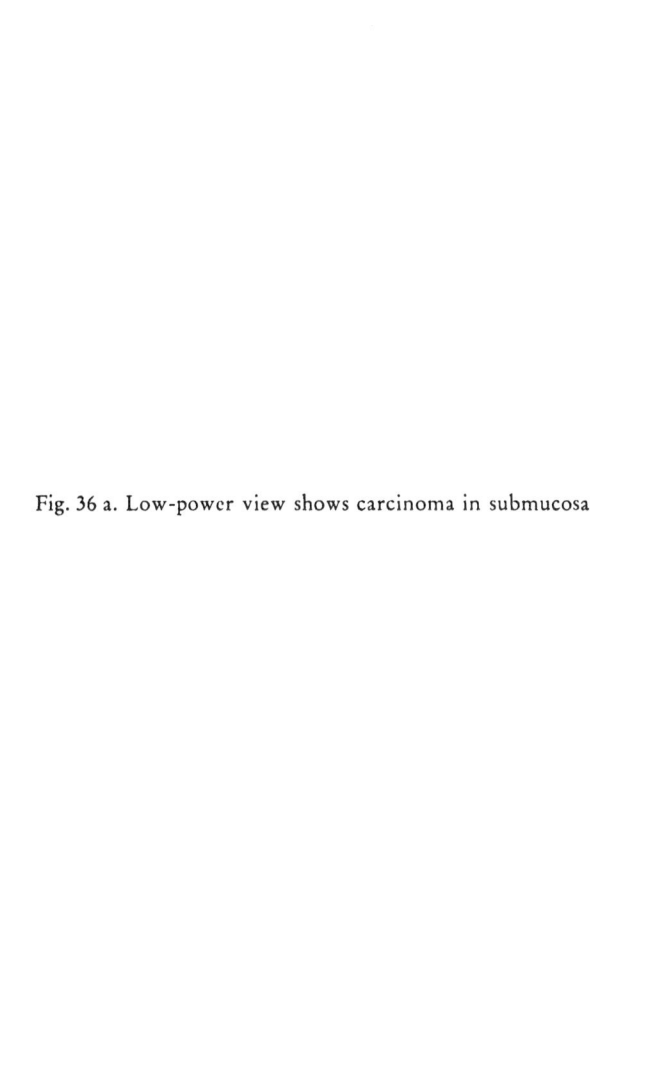

Fig. 36 a. Low-power view shows carcinoma in submucosa

Fig. 36 b. High-power view demonstrates signet-cell type of cancer

Fig. 37. A typical polypoid carcinoma is seen arising from the greater curvature and posterior wall of the antrum. It has a nodular surface, is more deeply red than the surrounding mucosa, and there is a small tumor component just proximal to the main mass

Fig. 38. A ring-shaped, submucosal carcinoma involves the antral canal. Distally, there is a nodular, irregular break in the ring, and blood may be seen running over the tumor to the left from its more necrotic interior

Fig. 39. The floor of the antrum is shown, with a peristaltic wave progressing distally. The anterior wall and adjacent greater curvature are involved with a flat, irregular, shallow ulceration beneath with there appears to be infiltration. This lesion proved to be a superficial carcinoma. There is little interference with peristalsis in the distal antrum

Fig. 40. Heavy, fixed folds of recurrent carcinoma are seen in the residual gastric pouch of a 29-year-old white woman who had had palliative resection for cancer of the stomach over four years previously. Chemotherapy was ineffective and she died with disseminated carcinomatosis

Fig. 41. This polypoid tumor was found on routine radiological follow-up in the residual gastric pouch of a patient who had had a curative resection for polypoid carcinoma of the stomach five years previously. At exploration the tumor was resected and proved to be carcinoma. All lymph nodes were negative, and he was alive and well two years later

Fig. 42. This projecting tumor was noted in the greater curvature of the antrum of a 65-year-old white man who had a large liver, proven by percutaneous liver biopsy to contain primary hepatoma. The whole floor of the antrum is deformed, and the black tumor mass appears to project from a craterlike elevation. At autopsy, it was found to consist of the primary liver tumor which had penetrated the stomach wall by direct extension

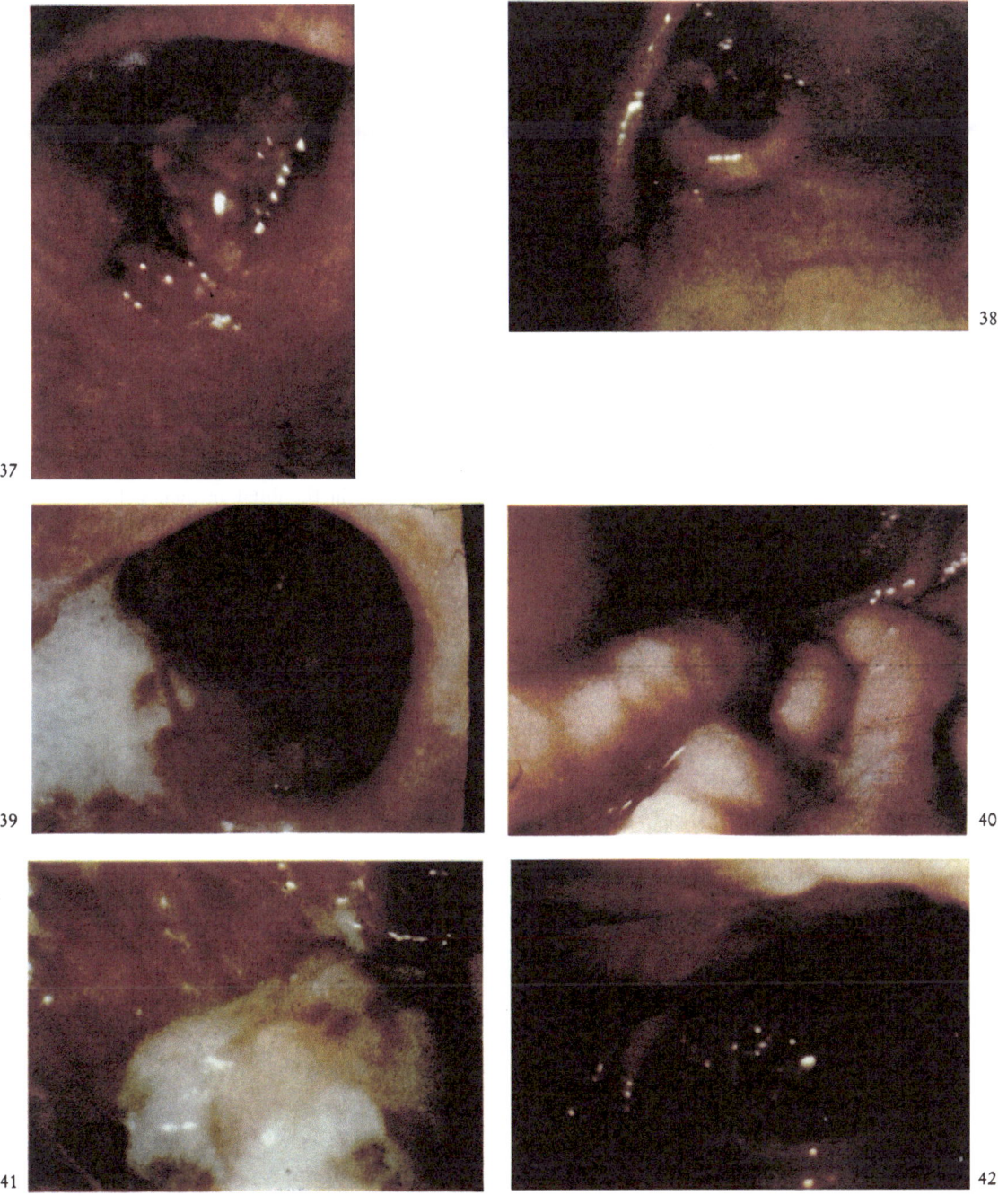

Fig. 43. This unique photograph was obtained in the stomach of a 34-year-old white man with biopsy proven malignant melanoma, involving skin, nodes and liver. His only gastrointestinal symptom was nausea, and roentgenograms had shown a normal stomach and a questionable duodenal nodule. The mucosa is studded with small black tumors, as shown by this view of the greater curvature of the antrum. Peristalsis was unimpeded

Fig. 44. A close-up view of the greater curvature of the body of the stomach shown in Fig. 43 demonstrates that the numerous nodules project above the mucosa like small polyps in some areas, and are smaller and more sessile in others

Fig. 45. The lesser curvature and antrum of this 63-year-old white woman, who had had nausea, vomiting, epigastric pain and melena for two months, is massively involved by tumor with rather bizarre characteristics. There is marked necrosis of the lesser curvature and anterior wall proximal to the antrum, a polypoid mass in the distal antrum, and a craterlike lesion on the proximal floor, with a similar, lower lesion laterally. The crater lesion has been quite characteristic of reticulum cell sarcoma in our series. Biopsy showed findings consistent with reticulum cell sarcoma (Fig. 45 a and 45 b), which was confirmed on autopsy three weeks later

Fig. 46. Massive submucosal tumor infiltrate observed in a 52-year-old woman with fever, weakness and epigastric distress. A biopsy taken through the esophagoscope showed reticulum cell sarcoma. Following radiation therapy to the stomach and lymph nodes, she did very well, and follow-up gastroscopy revealed essentially normal mucosa grossly and by biopsy

Fig. 47. Massive necrosis, ulceration and bleeding of the anterior wall and lesser curvature of the stomach is shown in a patient with reticulum cell sarcoma. The appearance improved somewhat following radiation, but the patient expired three months later

Fig. 48. Marked submucosal infiltration was found involving the stomach of this 42-ear-old white woman with biopsy proven (lymph nodes) lymphocytic lymphoma. A large doughnut-shaped lesion is seen in the distal antrum overriding the pylorus. Proximally, there are massive folds. She survived for two years following radiation therapy

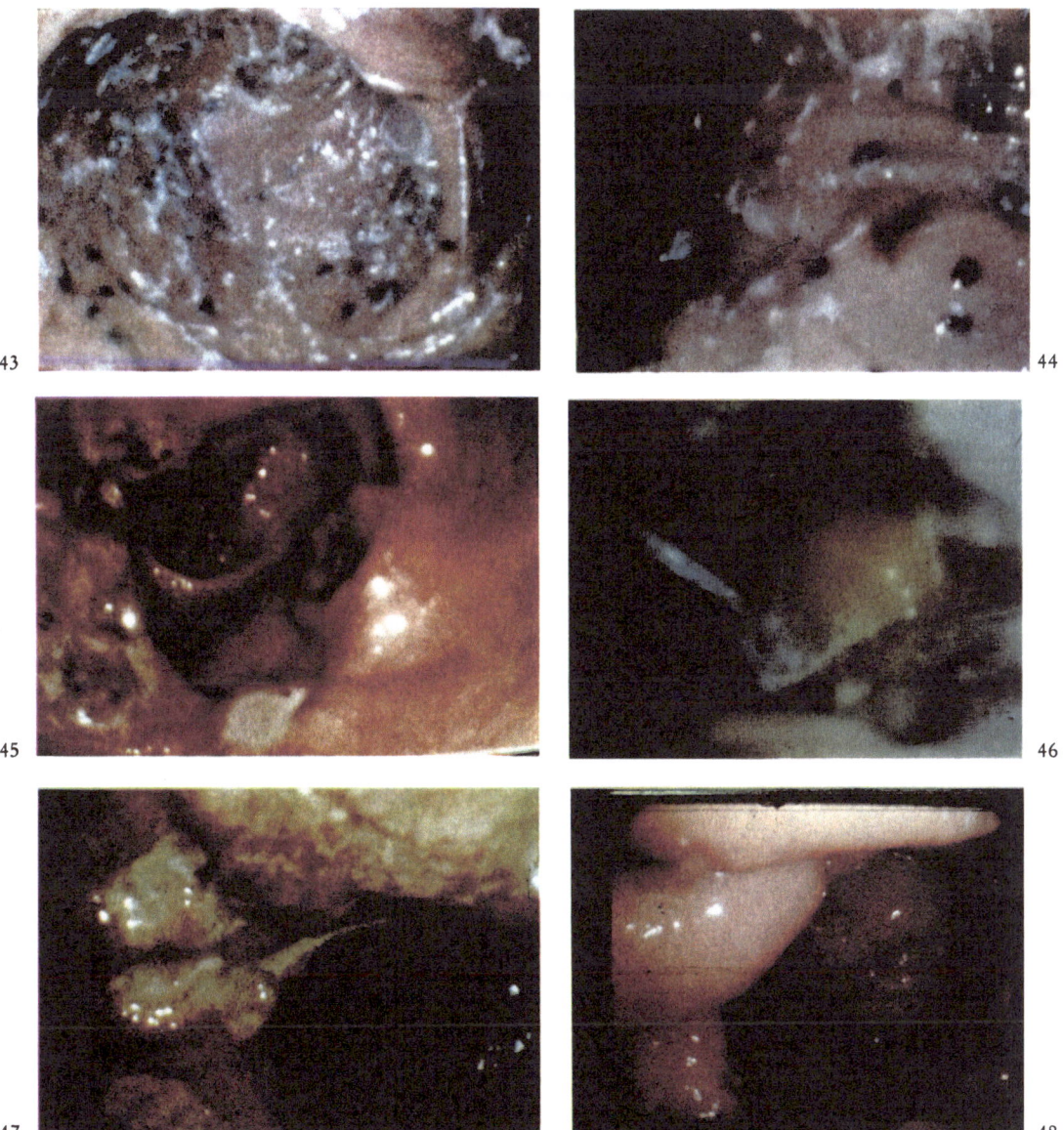

43

44

45

46

47

48

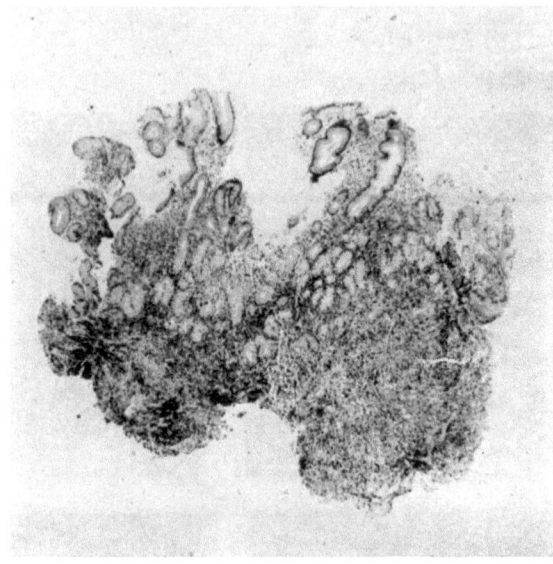

Fig. 45 a. Low-power view showing submucosal infiltrate of tumor cells (Fig. 45)

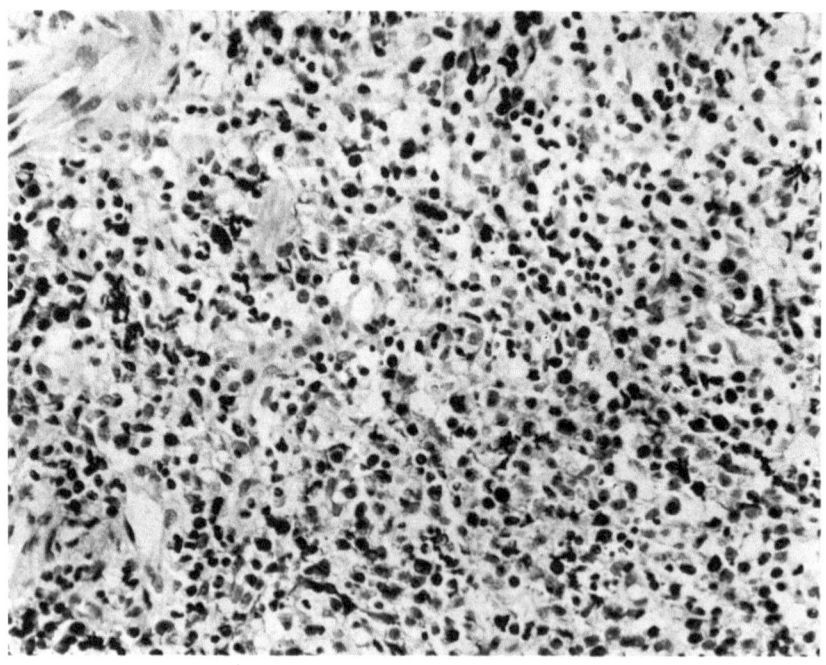

Fig. 45 b. High-power view of tumor infiltrate shown in Fig. 45 a

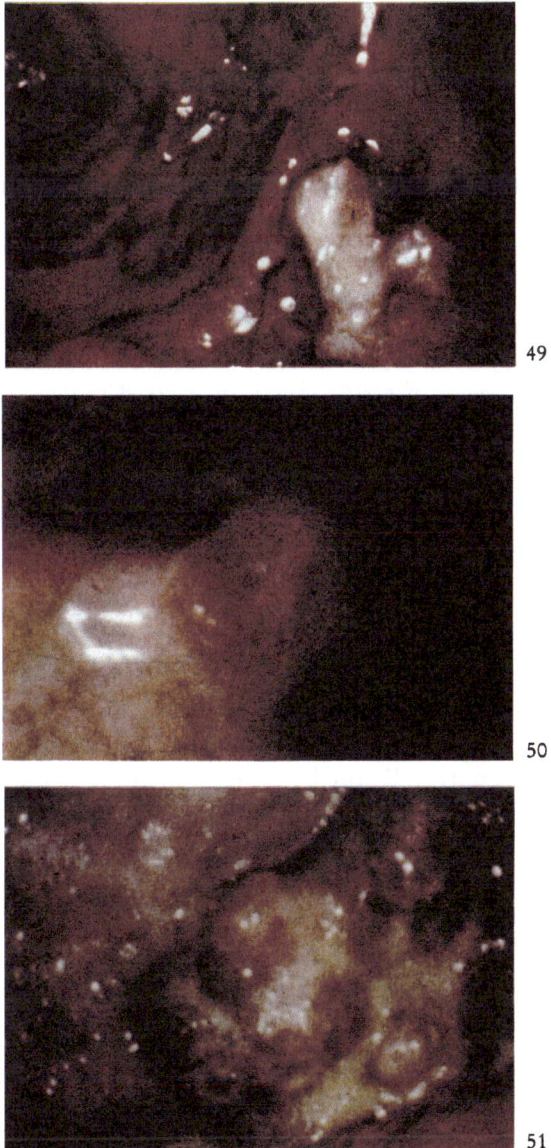

Fig. 49. Generalized swelling, infiltration, and a large flat ulceration of the posterior wall of the stomach are seen in this patient with lymphocytic lymphosarcoma

Fig. 50. A single, ulcerating, irregularly sharped polypoid nodule was noted on the greater curvature of the body of the stomach in this patient with proven multiple myeloma. Large nodular folds are shown progressing distally. At autopsy, myeloma infiltrates were found in the stomach wall

Fig. 51. A large meaty, nodular tumor mass is demonstrated in the remaining stomach pouch of a patient who had undergone previous subtotal gastric resection for a neurogenic sarcoma of the stomach. Besides the evident polypoid tumor there is suspicious change in the wall of the pouch laterally

Chapter 4

Endoscopy in Specific Clinical Situations

As one has the opportunity over the years to observe and evaluate many patients referred with the diagnosis of gastric cancer, or is asked to determine the cause of upper gastrointestinal complaints in patients with proven carcinoma elsewhere in the body, gastroscopy stands out in certain clinical situations as particularly rewarding. The totally roentgenographically-oriented physician, who is, one fears, in the majority, may never think to request the services of the gastroscopist when confronted with the situations to be described below, and it is for him that this particular chapter is written. He is, after all, the one who usually has first contact with the patient and his complaints, and if the description of a certain train of events strikes a chord and renders it possible to make an earlier diagnosis or to institute treatment more promptly in even a few cases, the purpose of this chapter will have been achieved.

Repeated Negative Radiological Examinations in the Face of Organic Symptoms

Strange though it may seem, relatively large carcinomas of the stomach may exist despite repeatedly negative roentgenograms. This happens, it is true, more frequently when the radiologist is inexperienced, or when interpretation of films, taken previously by technicians with less than average training and interest in their occupation, is attempted by "circuit riders", radiologists who make the rounds of outlying hospitals and clinics at intervals. Every year we see a few such patients, appearing with from two to four sets of stomach films, the last of which finally shows the tumor, now grown to such proportions that it is impossible for anyone to misinterpret the findings. In most of these situations, it appears probable that a more expert examination, including fluoroscopy, somewhere along the line, would have uncovered the pathology, and this is not an indictment of radiology. However, in a few cases, even expert radiologists, told in advance that gastroscopy had shown cancer, ulcer, or tumor, have been unable to demonstrate a lesion which was later found at surgery. The following report illustrates such a case, which was missed even at surgical exploration.

Case Report. This 59-year-old white male was first seen July 5, 1968 with a painful lump in the upper abdomen, marked weakness and loss of weight. Exploratory laparotomy had shown liver metastasis but the primary source of the tumor was not determined. A biopsy was taken which showed adenocarcinoma, metastatic to the liver. Repeated roentgenologic examinations showed hepatomegaly but no evidence of gastric pathology even after a tumor had been seen endoscopically. At gastroscopy a large ulcerating lesion with rolled cufflike edges was noted at the junction of the body of the stomach and antrum (Fig. 52). This was felt to be carcinoma with ulceration. The patient was placed on chemotherapy, and completed an initial course of 5-Fluorouracil but expired at home 3 months later.

Our radiologists, who are certainly expert, are aware of the possibility of missing lesions of the stomach, and also the advantages of an endoscopic examination when they sense there is something abnormal about a stomach, but cannot demonstrate it adequately. Consequently, we get many referrals which are stimulated by a request for gastroscopy from the radiologist himself. This type of cooperation has become standard in all institutions where there is a strong gastrointestinal endoscopy service (OLSEN, 1964), but unfortunately prevails almost nowhere else.

A more enlightened attitude concerning gastroscopy on the part of physicians who see patients with persistent, organic, undiagnosed abdominal pain would result in at least some decrease in morbidity.

Equivocal Radiologic Findings with or without Symptoms

Even more frequent than the negative radiological examination in the symptomatic patient is the situation in which the routine roentgenographic study results in equivocal findings possibly indicative of serious disease, or that in which the roentgenographic results in the symptomatic individual do not appear to fit the clinical picture, or at least require explanation.

An example is the 32-year-old man seen recently with a seven-day history of "heartburn". A routine x-ray examination was said to show a tumor of the fundus of the stomach. Careful gastroscopic survey of the entire gastric mucosa, including retroflexive visualization of the fundus, failed to reveal any abnormality. A repeat roentgenographic study by a different radiologist rendered the same findings, and the patient was not explored. He rapidly became asymptomatic on antacid and antispasmodic medication.

Another patient, a healthy-appearing woman in her forties, was referred by a surgeon who said he had had "three recent negative exploratory operations" on the basis of x-ray findings of a probable gastric tumor. Her gastroscopy was completely and unequivocally negative for pathology of any sort.

On the other hand, there may be legitimate roentgenographic abnormalities which are difficult to interpret. The following case reports illustrate such situations, all satisfactorily elucidated by gastroscopy.

Case Report. This 57-year-old surgeon was seen following an episode of massive upper gastrointestinal bleeding which had occurred immediately after a long and hazardous trip by automobile. X-ray examination had shown only a possible small prepyloric ulcer. At gastroscopy, a large benign-looking gastric ulcer, approximately 2 cm. in diameter, was noted on the lesser curvature side of the stomach (Fig. 53). The antrum appeared normal although there was hyperperistalsis. At subsequent gastroscopic examination three weeks later, the ulcer showed marked evidence of healing (Fig. 54) and two-and-a-half months later there was a complete healing of the lesser curvature ulcer. There was no evidence of recurrence during the next two years.

Comment: The convincing evidence, insofar as this physician patient was concerned, was the color photograph showing the large lesser curvature ulcer and normal, though hyperperistaltic antrum. He also appreciated follow-up pictures which demonstrated complete healing, and had no objection to undergoing gastroscopy three times in the process.

Case Report. A 67-year-old white male was admitted August 10, 1959 with a history of black tarry stools and abdominal swelling as well as abdominal cramps relieved by food. There had been a 15 pound weight loss but physical examination was essentially negative. Hemoglobin was 11.5 gms., white cells 5,950 with a normal differential, serology was negative, and stools positive for occult blood. Barium enema was negative. Upper gastrointestinal series on August 14, 1959, showed at least two rounded ulcerated masses in the stomach which had the appearance of leiomyoma or other intramural mass. The x-ray study was repeated four days later and the conclusion reached that there were multiple ulcerated polyps and intramural lesions of the stomach, the appearance of which was most suggestive of leiomyomata or neurofibromata. On August 20, 1959, gastroscopy revealed an ulceration of the posterior wall of the stomach but no definite tumor mass seen within the stomach itself. Ten days later gastroscopy was repeated because of the confusing x-ray report and the antrum ulceration was again visualized as well as a rather large persimmon bezoar in the midportion of the stomach resting on the greater curvature which subsequently rolled into the fundus (Fig. 55). The patient was advised to return to the hospital for surgery but failed to do so and follow-up letters were unanswered.

Comment: Bezoars are uncommon, but may be lethal (NELSON, 1963; PATTERSON and ROUSE, 1940; DE BAKEY and OCHSNER, 1939) as a result of ulceration and perforation. They do not, however, have the same connotation as cancer, and in one patient who had had a recent coronary occlusion, it was possible on the basis of the gastroscopic diagnosis to delay exploration until complete cardiac recovery had occurred.

Case Report. This 52-year-old white male was found to have multiple myeloma in December, 1968 when he consulted his physician for right lower chest pain of six weeks' duration. He was treated with Alkeran 6 mg. daily for 18 days. When first seen at The University of Texas M. D. Anderson Hospital, January 7, 1969, he was also found to have mild azotemia. He was treated with Melphalan 48 mg. daily for four days, and prednisone 120 mg. daily for nine days. A week after completion of this regimen, he noted a loss of appetite and inability to swallow large quantities of food at one time, and suffered a 20 pound weight loss over a period of three weeks. Roentgenograms showed an infiltrative lesion involving the greater curvature of the body of the stomach. Gastroscopy showed infiltrative submucosal tumor growth on the posterior wall of the body and fundus of the stomach, and directed biopsy was interpreted as adenocarcinoma of stomach, signet ring-cell type. He underwent total gastric resection, but did poorly and eventually expired.

Comment: The confusing finding of possible additional neoplasia in this patient with confirmed multiple myeloma could not be definitely substantiated by x-ray examination. A specific gross and histologic diagnosis was rendered by gastroscopy and biopsy within two days of referral.

Determination of Extent of Carcinomatous Involvement

In the early days of gastroscopy, it was hoped that it might be a means of accurate delineation of the gross involvement of the stomach in carcinoma. Due to the usual tendency of cancer to spread beyond the gastric wall, it was soon found that endoscopy would be only partially successful in preoperative evaluation. A fair approximation may be made, however, and gastroscopy may demonstrate more marked involvement of the mucosa than is revealed by x-ray examination, or delineate the intragastric spread more precisely, as in the following patient.

Case Report. A 75-year-old white male was seen with a main complaint of hematemesis and melena for 15 days. An ulcer had been noted on the previously obtained roentgenograms which were not available at the time of examination. Gastroscopy on July 1, 1969 showed a large ulcerating tumor mass which completely involved the antrum and partly encircled the stomach although the fundus itself seemed to be relatively uninvolved (Fig. 56). Biopsies taken from the tumor itself and the edge of the ulcer crater were read as showing adenocarcinoma of the stomach. Surgery was carried out one week later at which time a partial gastrectomy, omentectomy and gastrojejunostomy were performed for adenocarcinoma invading the full thickness of the gastric wall. Eight of 14 lymph nodes were positive. Five months later, he was doing well without evidence of metastatic disease.

Comment: Although the reported finding by x-ray was antral carcinoma, gastroscopy demonstrated, as frequently happens, that the tumor had spread along the lesser curvature of the body of the stomach. These findings were of some value to the surgeon prior to exploration.

Histologic Proof of Malignant Neoplasia in Poor Risk or Inoperable Patient Prior to Radiation or Chemotherapy

Gastroscopy may be the best means of obtaining histologic proof of cancer prior to institution of therapy in a patient who is a poor risk because of generalized debilitation or degenerative disease, or in the patient who has been previously explored with indeterminate results, in which a confirmed diagnosis is mandatory prior to radiation or chemotherapy. Gross and microscopic evidence may usually be obtained with a minimum of discomfort and risk, as described in the following instance.

Case Report. This 66-year-old white male began to have dull upper abdominal pain in March, 1969, followed after ten days by an episode of melena which made him feel quite weak. He was hospitalized and an exploratory laparotomy done on June 6, 1969 revealed a large tumor mass involving the posterior wall of the stomach. In addition, there were several large rounded tumor masses in the retroperitoneal area. Numerous enlarged lymph nodes were seen in the omentum, biopsy of which showed lymphosarcoma. (The official pathology report at M. D. Anderson Hospital was unclassified malignant neoplasm, histiocytic reticulum cell sarcoma being not excluded). The lesion was considered to be not resectable and the abdomen was closed.

At gastroscopy on June 26, 1969, a large fungating lesion involving the posterior wall, upper body and fundus was seen. The crater was very large, necrotic, and had a raised edge surrounding it. The area surrounding this lesion was also infiltrated with linear nodular infiltrate (Fig. 57). Biopsies showed unclassified malignant neoplasm (Fig. 57a).

He received XRT to abdomen (4000 rads in 5^1/$_2$ weeks) with considerable improvement. When seen in October, 1969, he had no abdominal symptoms and he felt quite well. Roentgenograms performed October 14, 1969 showed some distortion of the greater curvature of the gastric antrum but there was no definite evidence of tumor or ulceration. Gastroscopy on October 16, 1969 showed generalized mucosal atrophy and an area of converging folds on the posterior wall. Biopsy at this time showed no definite evidence of tumor.

Assessment of Results of Chemotherapy

Demonstration of the effects of chemotherapeutic agents in gastrointestinal cancer in general is very difficult. Objective evidence of antitumor action may be impossible to obtain, even when masses are available for measurement (MOERTEL and REITE-MEIER, 1969). In gastric cancer, it is possible in a small proportion of patients to obtain color photographs as well as biopsy specimens during the course of chemotherapy which objectively illustrate effective tumor suppression or insensitivity of the tumor to treatment. The number of such cancers will be small, however, since gross effects may be best determined in the polypoid or sharply delineated carcinomas, and only an occasional case will fit these criteria.

Recent reports (NELSON, 1969), show that this type of pictorial evidence of the results of therapy has become easier to obtain since the advent of the fiberscope-gastrocamera, and that the photographs are superior, although those taken with the older lens fiberscope and external camera were acceptable and useful (NELSON, 1963). From the clinical standpoint, treatment is particularly valuable in preventing obstruction in tumors of the antrum or cardia, or in preserving nutrition in advanced submucosal infiltrative lesions (linitis plastica).

Definitive results have been obtained with this method so far in 13 patients. Six showed measurable changes in intragastric carcinoma, in five the results were indeterminate, and in two there was obvious growth in the face of chemotherapy. Details of the evaluations of two patients are given below.

Case Report. A 45-year-old Spanish American male was seen March 6, 1968 with complaints of pain in the upper abdomen and heartburn over a period of 15 months. A recent biopsy of the supraclavicular nodes had shown metastatic carcinoma. An x-ray examination revealed a polypoid carcinoma of the stomach. At gastroscopy there was a very large polypoid lesion apparently attached on the posterior wall and lesser curvature side of the antrum (Fig. 58). Because of the metastatic disease, resection was not carried out and the patient was placed on 5-Fluorouracil on March 13, 1968. There was some evidence of necrosis as far as the tumor was concerned during follow-up but no real lessening in size (Fig. 59). He was last seen August 16, 1968 with evidence of liver metastasis and preterminal.

Comment: There was marked change in the polypoid mass under 5-Fluorouracil therapy, but follow-up photographs show at least as extensive involvement of the floor of the antrum as previously noted, and the overall result must be considered indeterminate.

Case Report. This 68-year-old white male was first seen December 27, 1967 following exploration for a perforated ulcer at which a large mass in the lower end of the stomach had been found and reported as poorly differentiated adenocarcinoma. Resection was not carried out. Roentgenogram showed an extensive carcinoma of the distal stomach with probable invasion of the pancreas and gastroscopic examination, carcinoma of the stomach involving the pylorus and antrum with a larger ulceration on the posterior wall (Fig. 60). Follow-up gastroscopic examinations following 5-Fluorouracil therapy showed considerable improvement in the appearance of the lesion (Fig. 61), the last endoscopy being performed November 12, 1968, nine months after the first. At that time very little change was noted but it was felt a good response had been obtained. The patient expired one month later of his disease, a little less than a year after first being seen.

Comment: The change in size and appearance of the lesion recorded in this patient is unequivocal. Not only is there marked improvement in both categories, but there is no evidence of further spread in the surrounding areas, as in the previous case.

Evaluation of Gastrointestinal Symptoms During Course of Known Cancer Elsewhere

Patients with known cancer, or those undergoing investigation for cancer, may develop upper gastrointestinal symptoms and signs which may or may not be related to neoplasia. These are sometimes the result of benign disease, but often signal the extension of malignancy to the stomach, or even the development of a second primary cancer. Regardless of the cause, it may denote disease quite as serious as the initial cancer, and complete and prompt evaluation is essential. Gastroscopy is frequently the most rapid and accurate means of determining the nature of new complications of this type.

Extension of known neoplasia and gastric ulceration are perhaps the commonest source of such symptoms under these circumstances. The following examples illustrate the role of gastroscopy in management.

Case Report. This 65-year-old colored man was first seen in November, 1968 for "lumps in the neck" of about six months' duration. He also complained of fever, sweating attacks and a weight loss of 30 pounds. Physical examination revealed massive lymphadenopathy in the neck, axillae and inguinal areas. Left axillary lymph node biopsy showed lymphohistiocytic proliferation with plasmocytosis. He was treated with chlorambucil and prednisone with some improvement and decrease in the size of lymph nodes.

In April, 1969, he complained of loss of appetite and epigastric fullness after meals. Roentgenograms showed marked hypertrophy of the mucosal folds in the stomach. Gastroscopy demonstrated submucosal nodular infiltrations both in the anterior and posterior walls at the beginning of the antrum. In addition, the mucosal folds in the antrum looked prominent (Fig. 62). Gastric biopsy from these nodules showed atypical lymphohistiocytic infiltration with plasmocytosis, the histological changes being similar to those seen in the lymph nodes previously (Figs. 62a and 62b). He continued to have fever, was placed on Leukeran and prednisone but did not respond and expired August 25, 1969. No autopsy was granted.

Comment: Roentgenoscopy can only point to the possibility of pathology when hypertrophied folds are the single finding. Gastroscopy allows a precise estimate as to involvement as well as a histological diagnosis.

Case Report. A 36-year-old white man was first seen July 28, 1969 with weight loss, lymphadenopathy, and abdominal cramps. Biopsy of nodes of the cervical region were interpreted as being amelanotic melanoma. Initial roentgenograms were read as showing no abnormalities but repeat examination revealed a 4 cm. in diameter irregular but well-defined mass on the greater curvature side of the stomach. Gastroscopic examination showed definite smooth submucosal infiltrations which were felt to represent malignant neoplasia (Fig. 63). This patient was biopsied on two occasions. On the second attempt, malignant tumor was found consistent with that removed from his cervical lymph nodes. He was placed on chemotherapy with some relief of symptoms and decrease in size of the peripheral metastatic lesions. Unfortunately, those in the stomach were not re-evaluated.

Comment: The initial x-ray examination in this case did show some suspicious irregularities, and in retrospect the diagnosis of normal stomach by the original radiologist seems unjustified. It was, however, accepted by the attending physician until gastroscopy showed tumor. This type of tumor, incidentally, may be quite difficult to biopsy, as was this one. The small biopsy forceps have a tendency to slide off the smooth, curved surfaces, since they have no cutting edge. The instrument fitted with a central needle to impale the tumor was finally successfully used to obtain an adequate biopsy in this patient.

Case Report. This 31-year-old white man, under investigation for undiagnosed cancer, and with a previous diagnosis of sequestration of the left lung with systemic aberrant arterialization and a left-to-right shunt was seen with massive hematemesis and melena. After preliminary gastric washing with saline, an ulcer was visualized on the posterior wall of the stomach but medial to this, there was an area of bright red bleeding with converging folds that appeared to be an ulcer crater hidden by the bleeding. The blood ran along the lesser curvature and dripped down in front of the scope (Fig. 64). Surgery was carried out within three days as an emergency revealing a massive lesser curvature peptic ulcer with active arterial bleeding. The ulcer was oversewn, and bilateral truncal vagotomy and pyloroplasty performed. He did quite well following this procedure except for some episodes of dumping syndrome.

Comment: Upper gastrointestinal bleeding constitutes a prime indication for endoscopy, especially in cancer patients on various types of therapy, who have their share of acute ulcerations and hemorrhagic gastritis, as well as esophagitis and esophageal varices. Arterial bleeding, as in this patient, usually obscures the actual ulcer crater, and secondary signs, such as converging folds, point to the pathology. Preparatory gastric lavage with iced saline is obligatory, and may still not dislodge large clots if they have formed.

Case Report. This middle-aged white male, who had had a carcinoma of the stomach removed by subtotal resection, developed epigastric pain and vomiting approximately one month post-operatively. Roentgenograms showed no definite pathology, but gastroscopy demonstrated the anastomosis clearly outlined with suture material, framing an edematous jejunum with an ulcer (Fig. 65). The patient did well following surgical correction.

Comment: Fiberoptic gastroscopy usually shows the gastroenterostomy and remaining gastric pouch to good advantage. Jejunal and anastomotic ulcerations are frequently missed by roentgenoscopy, due primarily to the rather high location of the gastric remnant which prevents palpation. In this case, it was possible to rule out missed tumor and point to the true, and correctible nature of the complication.

Pyloric Obstruction

Evidence of pyloric obstruction, usually obtained when barium is given to a patient with intractible vomiting, is often not satisfactorily explained by roentgenoscopy. The dilated, decompensated stomach, filled with the contrast media, seldom retains enough tone for the radiologist to outline the cause of obstruction at the pylorus. In such cases, after thorough washing and evacuation through a large gastric tube, endoscopy will in most instances show tumor if this is present. The procedure obviates the long period of nasogastric suction advocated by some as a means of determining the eventual course of action. The procedure and its advantages has been described in a previous report (NELSON and SIEGELMAN, 1965). An example of the employment of gastroscopy in this situation follows.

Case Report. This 74-year-old white female was first seen December 12, 1967 with a six months' history of nausea and vomiting. Roentgenograms showed a markedly dilated stomach filled with food, secretions and barium but no definite lesion could be seen because of the almost complete obstruction. Gastroscopy two days later showed a small hole representing the antral opening and massive submucosal tumor obstructing the antrum (Fig. 66). Palliative resection was carried out and the patient did fairly well until April 2, 1968 when she died of widespread gastric cancer.

Summary

The physician who is confronted with a patient with persistent organic upper gastrointestinal complaints cannot afford to accept persistently negative roentgenograms as proof that there is no lesion. Gastroscopy will in many instances assist in solving the problem. With established or suspected cancer, not all gastrointestinal complaints are related to the cancer, but may be caused by unsuspected benign disease, although there may also be extension to the stomach or a second gastric primary lesion. Endoscopy is a rapid and efficient means of making a precise diagnosis in many of such situations.

References

DeBakey, M., Ochsner, A.: Bezoars and concretions: a comprehensive review of the literature with an analysis of 303 collected cases and a presentation of eight additional cases. Surgery 4, 934 and 5, 132 (1939).

Nelson, R. S.: Gastroscopic observations on the persimmon bezoar. Bull. Gastroint. Endosc. 10, 9 (1963).

— Gastroscopic photography in the evaluation of cancer chemotherapy. Bull. Gastroint. Endosc. 10, 13 (1963).

— Lanza, F. L.: Gastroscopic color photography in cancer chemotherapy. Gastroint. Endosc. (in press).

— Siegelman, M. H.: Endoscopy in the management of pyloric obstruction. Amer. J. Gastroent. 44, 9 (1965).

Olsen, A. M.: In: Re Mine, W. H., Priestley, J. T., Berkson, J.: Cancer of the Stomach. Philadelphia (Pa.): W. B. Saunders Co. 1964, p. 43.

Patterson, C. D., Rouse, M. O.: Foreign bodies in stomach observed through the gastroscope. Texas St. J. Med. 36, 238 (1940).

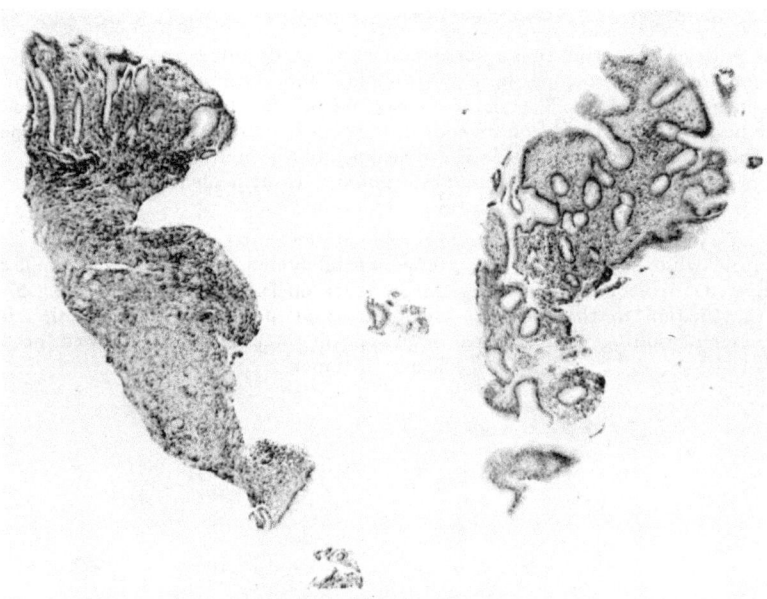

Fig. 57 a. Low-power view of gastroscopic biopsy from lesion in Fig. 57 demonstrating marked neoplastic invasion of the submucosa

Fig. 52. Several x-ray examinations and exploratory laparotomy at which this 59-year-old white man was found to have metastatic carcinoma of the liver had failed to reveal the primary tumor. Gastroscopy demonstrated a large ulcerating carcinoma of the lesser curvature and posterior wall high up on the body of the stomach. Following gastroscopy, the roentgenologist still could not find the lesion on careful examination

Fig. 53. A 52-year-old physician had suffered a massive upper gastrointestinal hemorrhage, and roentgenograms suggested the presence of a small antral ulcer. Gastroscopic photographs revealed a large benign-appearing ulcer of the lesser curvature and posterior wall. The contracting antrum, shown lateral to the ulcer, was not ulcerated

Fig. 54. After three weeks' medical therapy, the ulcer shown in Fig. 53 is approximately 20 per cent of its previous size. A final gastroscopy one month later revealed a normal stomach, and the patient has remained symptom-free for two years

Fig. 55. The photograph shows a black, apparently movable (proved by observation) rounded object lying in the mucus lake on the greater curvature of the fundus. The appearance is typical for persimmon bezoar, which in this patient was mistaken radiologically for cancer. When the patient stands up, the bezoar rolls to the antrum. Here, it was removed surgically and proved to be typical

Fig. 56. A large, ulcerating tumor surrounding and partly filling the antrum was seen and photographed at gastroscopy in a 75-year-old white man with a 15 day history of hematemesis and melena. The picture is taken from the level of the upper body, and it may be noted that the lesion extends upward along the lesser curvature and posterior wall. The fundus was uninvolved. The remainder of the mucosa shows atrophic changes, but is uninvolved. Biopsy was found to contain adenocarcinoma

Fig. 57. Very large, fixed, meaty-looking folds of the posterior wall of the stomach in a 66-year-old white male, whose enlarged peripheral lymph nodes showed lymphosarcoma on biopsy. Gastroscopic biopsy was interpreted as unclassified malignancy (Fig. 57 a). He received radiation to the abdomen, and gastroscopy performed four months after the initial examination revealed marked improvement. Repeat biopsy showed no definite evidence of tumor

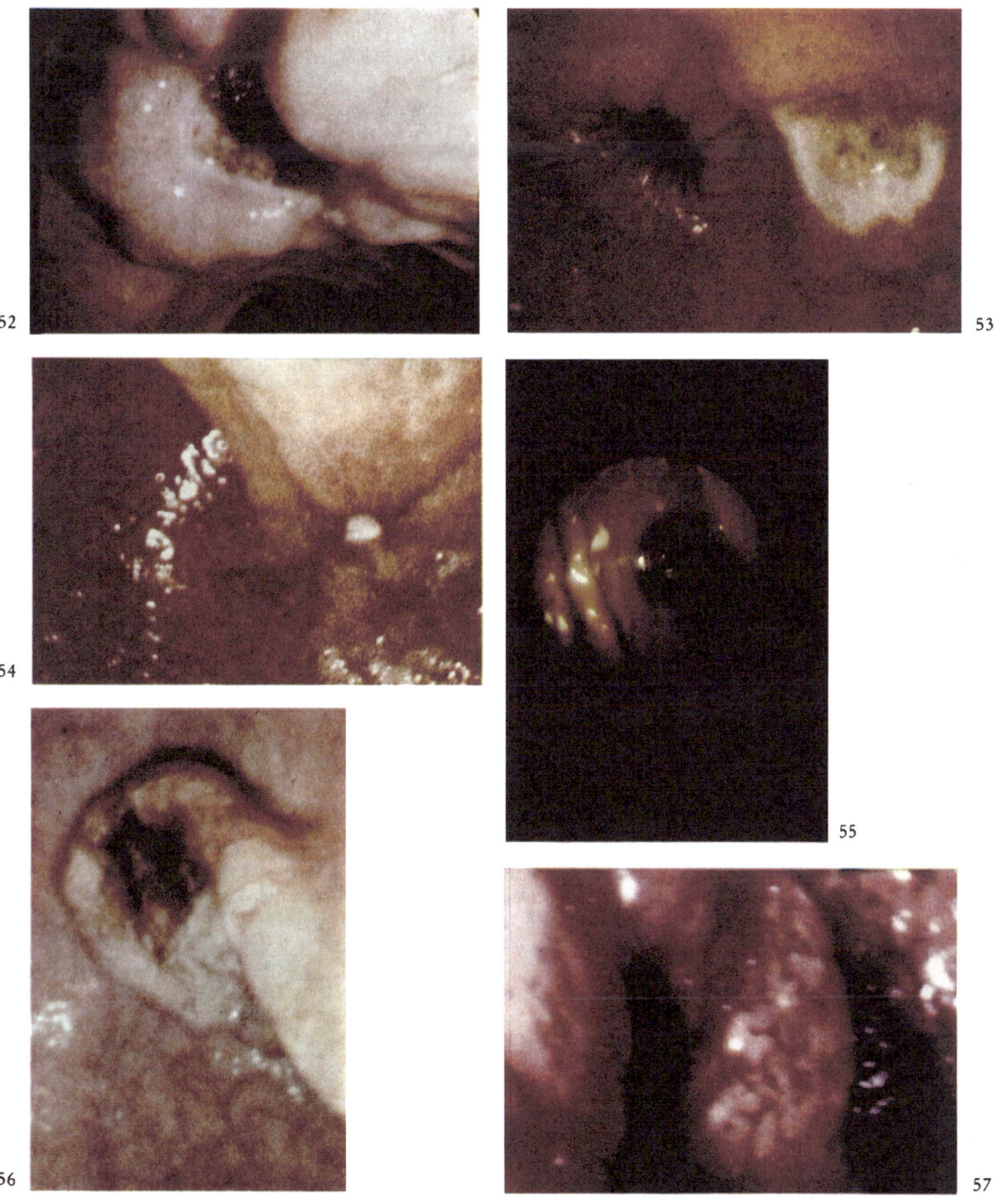

Fig. 58. A large polypoid carcinoma, apparently growing from the posterior wall and lesser curvature of the antrum, almost fills its lumen. The patient, a 45-year-old white man, had had epigastric pain and heartburn for 15 months, but no nausea or vomiting. A supraclavicular node was positive for adenocarcinoma

Fig. 59. Three months after the start of 5-Fluorouracil chemotherapy, the polyploid nature of the tumor (Fig. 58) has changed, and it now appears to invade the greater curvature and posterior wall of the antrum, with considerable necrosis. The antral canal may be seen distally, and there is still no obstruction

Fig. 60. A large ulcerating carcinoma involving the posterior wall of the antrum is shown, with marked necrosis. A strand of mucus extends across the entrance of the antrum to the anterior wall. The patient, a 67-year-old white man, had been previously explored and declared inoperable

Fig. 61. Following seven months of 5-Fluorouracil therapy, the lesion shown in Fig. 60 has decreased markedly in size, and is now represented by a localized ulceration of the posterior wall of the antrum, with minimal infiltration

Fig. 62. This view, taken into the antrum from the mid-portion of the stomach, demonstrates a large, club-like, infiltrated fold on the anterior wall, extending up to a thickened lesser curvature. Large folds are also noted proximally involving the anterior wall. The patient, a 65-year-old white man, complained of weight loss, fever, and lymphadenopathy, biopsy of which was designated as "lympho-histiocytic proliferation of plasma cell infiltration, suggesting a dysproteinemic process". Gastroscopic biopsy of the enlarged, club-like fold demonstrated essentially the same process (Fig. 62 a and 62 b)

Fig. 63. Large nodular tumor masses (two) are seen superimposed on the posterior wall of the stomach in a patient with proven metastatic amelanotic melanoma. Gastroscopic biopsies revealed the same tumor

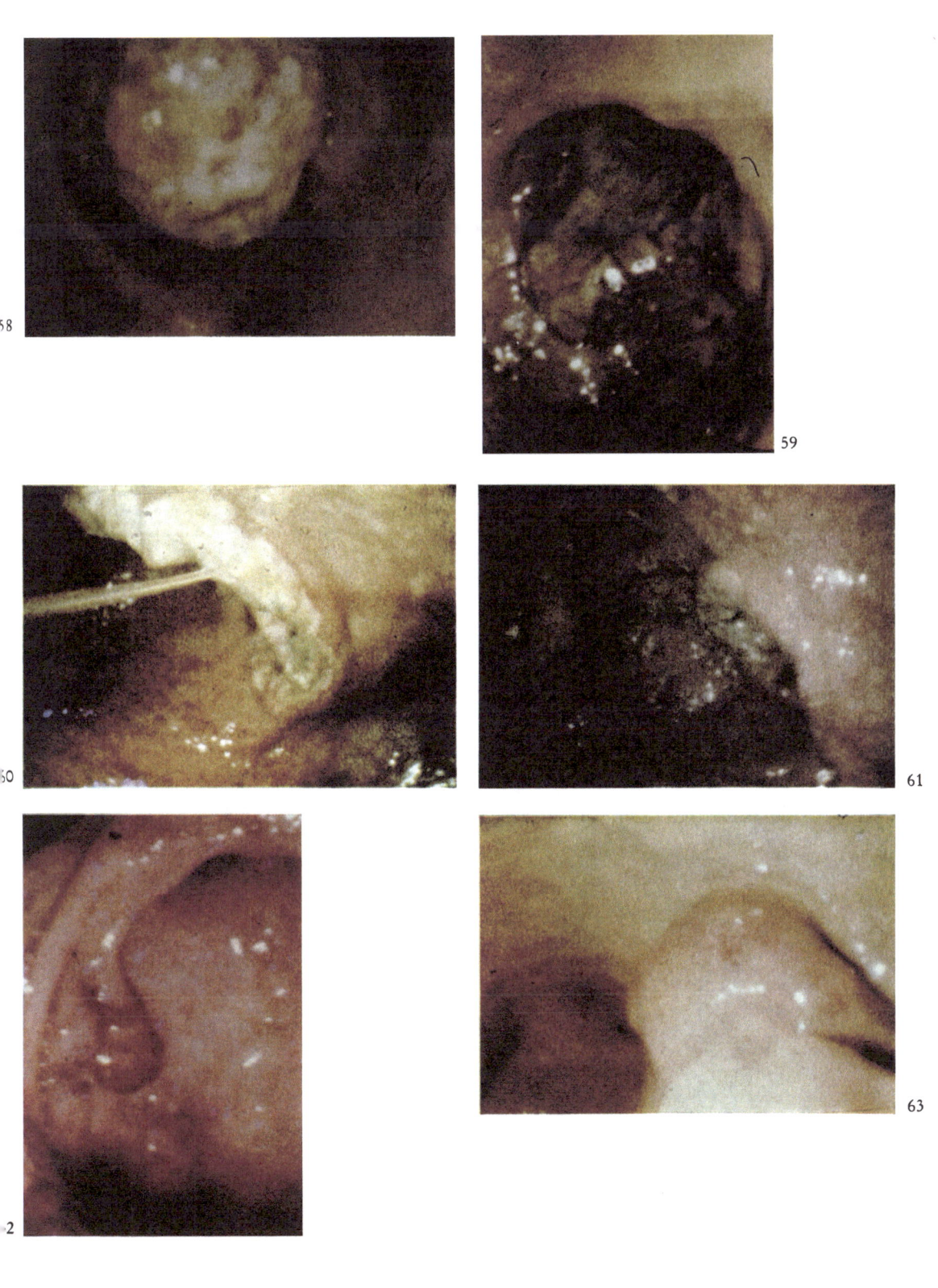

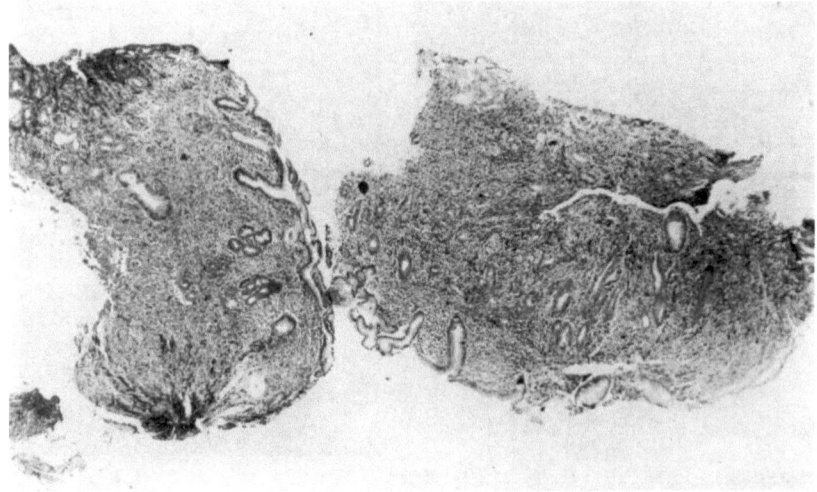

Fig. 62 a. Low-power view demonstrating abnormal mucosa and massive neoplastic infiltrate

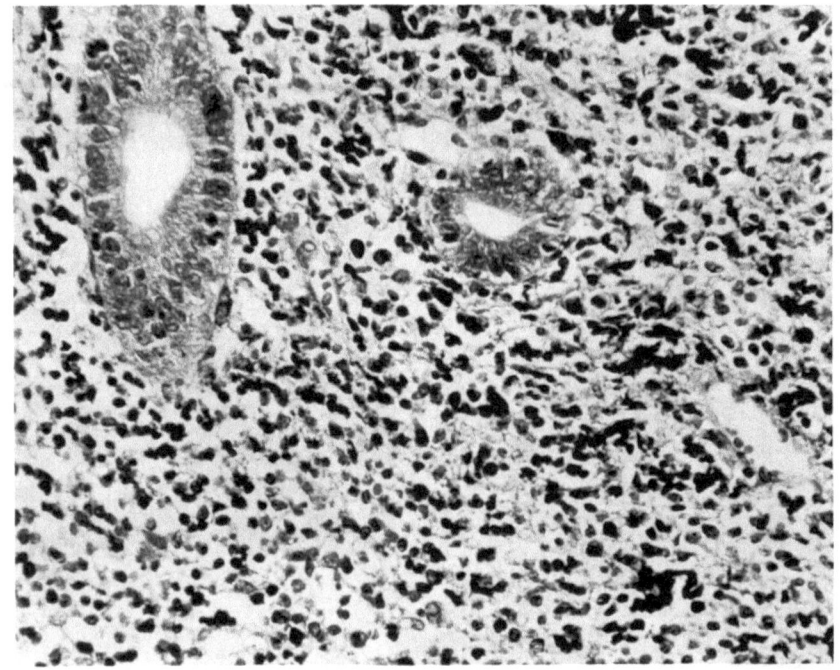

Fig. 62 b. High-power view of infiltrated area

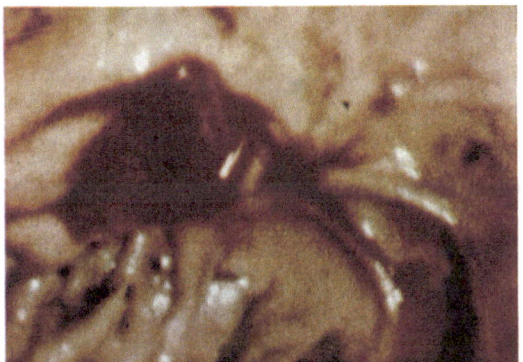

Fig. 64. This photograph shows rapid arterial bleeding in the stomach, determined at surgery as coming from an acute gastric ulcer. Although the crater cannot be seen, the main point of bleeding was noted to be at the convergence of who folds which are visible coming to a point on the lesser curvature. The blood seen proximally was noted at gastroscopy to be running along the lesser curvature and dripping down in front of the objective. The mucosa is pale, and clotted blood may be seen in the folds

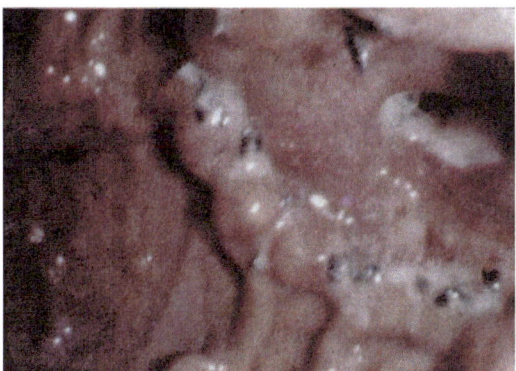

Fig. 65. This photograph was taken in the gastric pouch of a patient following subtotal resection for carcinoma who developed epigastric pain. The roentgenogram was indeterminate. The anastomosis can be seen, neatly outlined by suture material. This frames the markedly edematous jejunal mucosa (upper right) which is the seat of a benign-looking ulceration, confirmed at re-exploration

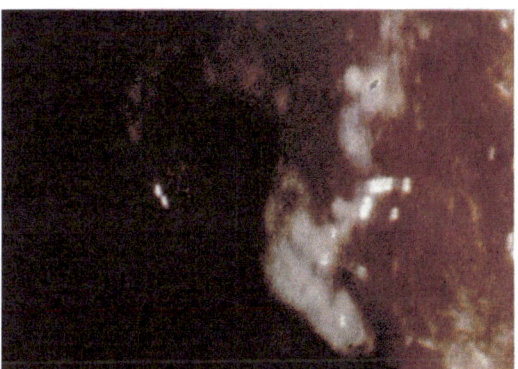

Fig. 66. The protruding, infiltrated area shown in this photograph represents all that is left of the antrum of a 74-year-old white woman who had a six months' history of nausea and vomiting. Roentgenograms showed only a barium filled stomach. Remains of the antral canal are represented by the dark hole in the center of the mass, proven at exploration to be adenocarcinoma

Chapter 5

The Future Relationship of Endoscopy to Gastric Cancer

The rapid changes which have taken place in the gastroscopic method during the past 10 years, which have amounted to a small revolution, are bound to have an effect on the diagnosis and management of gastric cancer in the years ahead. The magnitude of this effect, and whether the rapid advances will be suitably assimilated and adequately exploited, depend upon a number of factors. These are in most instances not directly related to the improvement in gastroscopic instruments already achieved and those to come, although this improvement also plays a part.

The endoscopist (and as he often suspects, the patient) has been handicapped in the past by infrequent resort to gastroscopy. So far as the gastroscopist is concerned, his experience leads him to believe that this inadequate use of a valuable method is more due to physician than patient resistance. The same doctor who will refer a patient for sigmoidoscopy without a second thought shies away from the suggestion of gastroscopy as though some unthinkable ordeal was intended. Yet for some years, almost every patient on our service who has had both types of endoscopy, when questioned, has admitted that he had less discomfort from gastroscopy than sigmoidoscopy. Even some endoscopists who apparently have a high regard for the procedure list, in their writings, so many contraindications as to limit the eligible list to a negligible few. One of these authorities (JOHNSON, 1951) lists no less than 15 such situations, only three or four of which we would consider as risky. A typical example is the old-age debilitated individual, a group which comprises a majority of gastric cancer patients on our service, and indeed a fair proportion of all those undergoing gastroscopy in our hospital. We have found debilitated old age, per se, not even a relative contraindication; in fact, the older patients, most of whom have a fairly philosophical outlook, usually are most cooperative and appreciative, even on repeated examination. Their complications are no more frequent than in the young and vigorous.

The time has come for an overhauling and reappraisal of all old ideas and conceptions in gastroscopy. Where it applies to cancer, this need for re-evaluation is urgent. The gastroscopist-oncologist is not so naive as to believe that application of this method on a wide scale would make a great improvement in cancer mortality. However, he cannot help have faith that it would decrease morbidity in many patients in a disease which has resisted all efforts to produce some kind of diagnostic and therapeutic breakthrough.

Future Instrument Development

Improvement in gastroscopes has always been limited by the anatomy of the organ to be viewed, particularly its proximal opening, the cardia. This allows one to pass an instrument of a relatively small diameter, in which must be included a number of systems for lighting, tip control, biopsy, and in some cases, photography. There is no gastroscope at present which can include the optimally-useful device for each of these purposes, even though some come close.

It has been stated previously (Chapter 11) that color photography and biopsy are the two features of the modern fibergastroscope which have been most valuable in the development of gastroscopy. Our experience would lead us to believe that the best still photographs will probably be obtained with the intragastric gastrocamera as part of a fibergastroscope, but it is impossible to incorporate this camera and a biopsy apparatus in the same instrument. On the other hand, fiberoptic lighting has improved photography with the external camera to such a degree that excellent color pictures, both still and cine, are now being obtained with this type of equipment. In the diagnosis of cancer, at least, biopsy has at last become very important to gastroscopists, and the instrument for this purpose should probably be one with biopsy potential, fiberoptic lighting, and external camera.

The ultimate instrument, and the one to which all present roads in fiberoptics seem to be leading, is the universal fiberscope, with forward viewing, fiberoptic lighting, controllable tip, and external camera. This will be long enough so that at the same procedure the esophagus, stomach, and hopefully part of the duodenum may be viewed in sequence. The only possible question is whether the forward-viewing feature will be as efficient as the present side-viewing fibergastroscopes to which we have all become accustomed. Preliminary tests with early models such as the Olympus Fiber Esophagoscope EF and ACMI Universal indicate that they probably will be, although it appears that inflation may be somewhat more difficult, and that clearing of the objective of mucus and debris will be more of a problem than with an instrument which can be wiped off by rotation against the mucosa.

Gastroscopists can confidently look forward to an instrument of this type. It should decrease costs by eliminating the necessity of maintaining a whole cabinet of different gastroscopes and esophagoscopes, and save time and discomfort for the patient. Although many of the oldsters (the author included) will probably resort to his favorite rigid esophagoscope or gastrocamera-fiberscope from time to time, or occasionally find a situation in which a plain fiberoptic, side-viewing biopsy gastroscope seems more appropriate, this combination instrument appears to be the endoscope of the future for the upper gastrointestinal tract, as does a similar device for the lower colon and rectum (presently available from Olympus Corporation).

Improvement in Procedure

The completely fiberoptic instruments have improved the gastroscopic examination for the patient in every way. During the procedure, he usually can lie in sedated ease with the flexible tube protruding in much the same manner as in gastric analysis, but with more comfort, due to the medication. Sedation has also been improved. Some gastroscopists now routinely employ intravenous valium (diazepam), which produces drowsiness without complete unconsciousness, and apparently amnesia for the period of sedation in a certain number (TICKTIN and TRUJILLO, 1968). Intravenous demerol (meperidine) is regularly given by others, with apparently equally good results. Local anesthesia has been abandoned entirely as unnecessary by some operators, although we still find it worthwhile.

Besides providing color records of pathology, fibergastroscopes have also aided in teaching by allowing the operator to bend the proximal end of the instrument and the ocular around so that all observers may have a view without disturbing the patient. In addition, one manufacturer provides a fiberoptic extension of the instrument for an additional viewer while the gastroscopist proceeds with the examination.

Despite the added patient comfort and definite teaching advantages, surveys reveal that the fibergastroscopes have a slightly higher incidence of perforation and mortality than their older lens counterparts. Comparison of a study by PALMER and WIRTS (1957) with a later survey by KATZ (1969), showed that of 267,175 gastroscopies with the semi-flexible lens gastroscope, 163 had perforations (.061%) with an overall mortality of 38 (.014%), while there were 24 perforations in 32,237 examinations with the fibergastroscope (.074%), and an overall mortality of six (.019%). The difference is not statistically significant, but points up the fact that any endoscope may be dangerous on occasion, especially in inexpert hands, or when used with the assumption that it is "safe". As pointed out by PALMER (1969), the original fibergastroscope was marketed with the claim that it was "100 per cent flexible and, therefore, completely safe." All such instruments have a rather large, rigid head, and perforations may be produced with them despite their flexibility. They should be introduced and manipulated with the same care as the older lens models. This part of modern procedure has not changed, and undoubtedly never will. The continued danger (although admittedly small) points up the necessity for proper training in endoscopy.

Expanded Training for Endoscopists

The correct method of endoscopic training has always been the subject of considerable debate. The best time to acquire such skills appears to be during the period of gastrointestinal residency or fellowship. Whether it will be provided during such training, however, depends on the orientation of the particular institution involved. Some gastroenterology services depend little on endoscopy and lean much more to basic research. Later on in practice, the graduate of these institutions may acquire an interest in endoscopy and wish to obtain some training.

A second group comprises those graduate physicians whose interest in gastroenterology began while in practice. Most of these, in our experience, have been internists, with a scattering of surgeons. These also should have an opportunity to learn.

The institution providing training in gastroscopy and other forms of gastrointestinal endoscopy should probably, therefore, provide programs for both of these groups. Although it is obvious that the time available for residents and fellows will be considerably greater than for the graduate physician who must in most cases continue to practice as he learns, programs may be devised to give adequate opportunities for both groups.

It is our belief, strengthened by experience over the past 20 years, that there is no short cut to gastroscopic or other endoscopic training. To be effective, it must include the personal performance of procedures, under expert supervision, in a fairly large number of patients, who should be picked to exhibit all possible types of pathology. This is a time-consuming and often tedious duty for the instructor, but unless he is willing to put forth the effort, he should not teach. Any short 10 to 14 day period of instruction, with the personal performance of four or five gastroscopies, is really orientation, and should not form the basis for purchase of a gastroscope and solo gastroscopy.

The first requisite for training in gastroscopy is therefore an institution with a service on which a large number—preferably 300 to 400—procedures are done yearly, headed by an enthusiastic and expert teacher of endoscopy. Clinics should be held two or three times weekly, with adequate time for complete evaluation of patients and instruction of the student, ordinarily the residents or fellows, who should each have his share.

The training of graduate physicians in such an institution is a far more difficult matter, and the decision to give courses of this type should not be taken lightly, as it entails a great deal of work and organization. Our approach has been to take one such student at a time, once weekly, for a period of six months. His training during each weekly session is essentially that of the resident, and care must be taken that the advancement of the latter is not jeopardized in the process. Because of the difficulty of arranging this type of instruction, we have not advertised these courses. They are listed by the postgraduate school, and all inquiries are referred to the dean. If the prospective student will agree to the times of attendance, however, and appears to be an honest prospect, every effort is made to accommodate him. The graduates are not finished gastroscopists, but most of them have used their knowledge and become excellent endoscopists with a minimum of patient trauma. There undoubtedly are other approaches to the problem of postgraduate endoscopic training, but we feel that for the individual who expects to wield a gastroscope, less time and effort than that described is useless.

Other short postgraduate courses, such as those sponsored in 1966 and 1969 by the American Society for Gastrointestinal Endoscopy (ASGE) are, however, very useful and have been extremely well attended. The latter of these two, held in Washington, D. C., had 486 registrants, and another 100 persons could not be accommodated because of lack of space. Since this number is close to double the membership of the ASGE, it appears obvious that many gastroenterologists are interested in endoscopy. The growing numbers of ASGE members also attest to this fact. This should be clear evidence that endoscopic training is important to the younger physician and should be provided at the residency level in all teaching institutions. The courses provided, we believe, would best be guided by the principles described in this section. If possible, where there is a demand, adequate training should also be available for a limited number of selected postgraduate students.

6*

Improved Orientation of the Physician Public

Most specialists are at least aware of the possible advantages of gastroscopy, and occasionally avail themselves of the services of an expert endoscopist when confronted with a difficult problem. The general practitioner, however, is often unaware that he has any recourse to definitive examinations other than roentgenoscopy in the patient with unexplained upper gastrointestinal symptoms and negative roentgenograms. Yet he is the one who has first contact with the problem, on whose shoulders lies the responsibility for further investigation under such circumstances. It is the clear duty of all gastroenterological endoscopists to publicize the advances in gastroscopy, particularly its expanded usefulness in the diagnosis and management of gastric cancer.

A good many papers are being presented on this subject these days, and like many other topics, are receiving a certain amount of publicity in the lay press. Additional reviews appear from time to time in the myriad of unofficial medical publications with which the physician is besieged through the mails. The ASGE has its own quarterly journal "Gastrointestinal Endoscopy," which is more or less unique, except for some Japanese publications, in devoting its contents almost exclusively to the subject. The standard medical journals also contain material of this type from time to time. However, some doctors apparently remain uninformed, and some of the informed remain unconvinced.

The best publicity for gastroscopy is undoubtedly the solution, at the grass roots level, of some knotty clinical problem for a specific physician, who then becomes convinced of the value and uses of the method. This gradual, slow but thorough type of education is probably the best source of referral for gastroscopic examination. It behooves all endoscopists to do their share in training of other physicians to perform gastroscopy, to keep themselves current on the latest advances and techniques, to be available to perform the procedure whenever asked, and to provide their share of sober publicity at the local level of state and county medical society meetings. There is plenty to talk about in the endoscopic line these days, and it should be widely presented.

The Gastroscopic Contribution to Improvement in Morbidity and Mortality in Gastric Cancer

The natural course of gastric cancer being what it is, there will undoubtedly be a considerable time lag before the exact contribution of endoscopy to the problem can be determined, even in Japan, where tremendous efforts at diagnosis have uncovered large numbers of patients early in the disease in time for definitive surgery (Chapter 2). At present, we have no means of knowing how many of such patients represent invasive cancer, and how many the early metaplasia usually labelled as carcinoma-in-situ. Conceding that all patients in whom a diagnosis of early disease has been made represent the former, it may still be unclear as to how many of these are cured by early surgery. We see relatively few patients with early lesions at The University of Texas M. D. Anderson Hospital and Tumor Institute, but the results in several of these, in whom curative resections were performed which yielded no positive nodes or serosol involvement, have been discouraging enough to warrant caution in prognosis, if the patient is followed over a sufficiently long period.

Two of these are worth describing in detail. One, a Latin-American man who underwent subtotal resection for a non-healing gastric ulcer which was determined to have minimal carcinomatous infiltration in the submucosa only, was followed for a period of four and one-half years, was asymptomatic, and eventually ceased to keep his appointments because he felt perfectly well. Nine and one-half years later he appeared in the clinic with ascites. Roentgenograms and endoscopy showed almost complete occlusion of the gastric pouch with tumor, a rectal shelf, and invasion of the large bowel. He died six months later despite chemotherapy. The second, a man in his middle sixties, had a carcinomatous ulcer removed without evidence of nodal or serosal spread. He was lost to follow-up for 10 years, and then appeared complaining of "bone pain." A roentgenographic skeletal survey showed multiple metastases, and biopsy revealed adenocarcinoma. Postmortem examination some weeks later confirmed the diagnosis of recurrent gastric carcinoma.

It has long been clear to those who follow long-term survivals from gastric cancer that this does not depend upon the resectability of the tumor in all cases, and palliative surgery will yield an occasional 10-year survivor. Five-year survivals may not be too significant. The uncertain prognosis despite the lack of evidence of metastases in some patients must give pause to those who might claim that all early cancer is "cured" if we can but get the patient to the radiologist or endoscopist early enough.

There is, however, no reason for a defeatist attitude. At the very least, the individual patient will suffer much less morbidity with prompt treatment of his cancer in a resectable stage. At the best, the early diagnosis of gastric cancer by all means including endoscopy, which we believe should now play a major role, will improve the mortality figures from this disease in future years.

Summary

Advances in gastroscopy have been so considerable as to call for a complete re-evaluation of indications and attitudes towards this procedure. Future instruments will in all probability be more efficient and designed for universal employment in esophagus, stomach, and duodenum. Improvements in anesthesia and technique have also taken place making the procedure more acceptable. Endoscopic training is still a problem, and should be made more generally available by teaching institutions. The physician public, meanwhile, must be educated to request gastroscopy more frequently in difficult diagnostic problems involving the stomach. Endoscopy may not, in the long run, make major improvements in the mortality from gastric cancer, but will reduce morbidity and aid greatly in the management of the individual patient.

References

JOHNSON, T. A.: Gastroscopy and gastric surgery. S. Clin. North. Amer. **31**, 651 (1951).

KATZ, D.: Morbidity and mortality in standard and flexible gastrointestinal endoscopy. Gastroint. Endosc. **15**, 134 (1969).

PALMER, E. D.: Discussion. Gastroint. Endosc. **15**, 141 (1969).

— WIRTS, C. W.: Survey of gastroscopic and esophagoscopic accidents. Report of committee on accidents of the American Gastroscopic Society. J. Amer. med. Ass. **164**, 2012 (1957).

TICKTIN, H. E., TRUJILLO, N. P.: Further experience with diazepam for pre-endoscopic medication. Gastroint. Endosc. **15**, 91 (1968).

Monographs already Published

27 SZYMENDERA, J., Warsaw: Bone Mineral Metabolism in Cancer. DM 32,—;
    US $ 8.80
28 MEEK, E. S., Bristol: Antitumour and Antiviral Substances of Natural Origin.
    DM 16,—; US $ 4.40
29 Aseptic Environments and Cancer Treatment. Edited by G. MATHÉ, Villejuif
    (Symposium). DM 22,—; US $ 6.10
30 Advances in the Treatment of Acute (Blastic) Leukemias. Edited by G. MATHÉ,
    Villejuif (Symposium). DM 38,—; US $ 10.50
31 DENOIX, P., Villejuif: Treatment of Malignant Breast Tumors: Indications and
    Results. DM 48,—; US $ 13.20
32 NELSON, R. S., Houston: Endoscopy in Gastric Cancer. DM 48,—; US $ 13.20

    Special Supplement: Biology of Amphibian Tumors. Edited by M. MIZELL,
    New Orleans. DM 86,—; US $ 24.00

In Production

33 Experimental and Clinical Effects of L-Asparaginase. Edited by E. GRUND-
    MANN, Wuppertal-Elberfeld, and H. F. OETTGEN, New York (Symposium).
    DM 58,—; US $ 16.—
34 ENDO, H., Fukuoka, T. ONO, Tokyo, T. SUGIMURA, Tokyo: Chemistry and
    Biological Actions of 4-Nitroquinoline 1-oxide

In Preparation

ACKERMANN, N. B., Boston: Use of Radioisotopic Agents in the Diagnosis of
Cancer

BOIRON, M., Paris: The Viruses of the Leukemia-sarcoma Complex

CAVALIERE, R., A. ROSSI-FANELLI, B. MONDOVI, and G. MORICCA, Roma: Selec-
tive Heat Sensitivity of Cancer Cells

CHIAPPA, S., Milano: Endolymphatic Radiotherapy in Malignant Lymphomas

Cutane paraneoplastische Syndrome. Edited by J. J. HERZBERG, Bremen
(Symposium)

GRUNDMANN, E., Wuppertal-Elberfeld: Morphologie und Cytochemie der Car-
cinogenese

IRLIN, I. S., Moskva: Mechanisms of Viral Carcinogenesis

LANGLEY, F. A., and A. C. CROMPTON, Manchester: Epithelial Abnormalities
of the Cervix Uteri

MATHÉ, G., Villejuif: L'Immunothérapie des Cancers

NEWMAN, M. K., Detroit: Neuropathies and Myopathies Associated with
Occult Malignancies

OGAWA, K., Osaka: Ultrastructural Enzyme Cytochemistry of Azo-dye Carcinogenesis

PARKER, J., and R. J. LUKES, Los Angeles: Lymphocyte Transformation in
Neoplastic Disease

PENN, I., Denver: Malignant Lymphomas in Transplant Patients

WEIL, R., Lausanne: Biological and Structural Properties of Polyoma Virus and
its DNA

WILLIAMS, D. C., Caterham, Surrey: The Basis for Therapy of Hormon Sensi-
tive Tumours

WILLIAMS, D. C., Caterham, Surrey: The Biochemistry of Metastasis